50 GEOMETRIC MANDALAS VOL 1

Easy to complex designs with notes, quotes and jokes for both kids and adults to color

✓ A Jumbo 50 Geometric Mandala designs - favourites for those who love coloring form and designs.

✓ The opposing pages to the designs have a quotes, interesting facts or jokes all the family will enjoy.

✓ Designs allow for both simple and advanced color blending, depending on your level of experience.

✓ This supports your natural growth as a coloring hobbyist – for both children and adults.

✓ A great form of art therapy to help you deal with anxiety, stress, just feeling low or even anger.

✓ You can taste and feel: calmness, creativity, joy, satisfaction, stress relief, fun, mindfulness and a sense of achievement.

✓ Sharing with your spouse, partner, children or grandchildren enhances both the creative experience and your relationships.

HEY THERE! COLOR ME TOO

1

Register – it's FREE - for our Insider's Club and get a pdf of coloring pages at
www.DancingWithYourLife.com
And check out the full range of our books and products while you're there.

****

2

Send us a photo of your proudest colored page from one of our coloring books. The best ones selected each month will be posted on our web site. These winners will get their choice of a free coloring book
Email: support@DancingWithYourLife.com

****

3

Please leave a review to let us know how you went with this book at:
www.amazon.com/gp/product/994423047

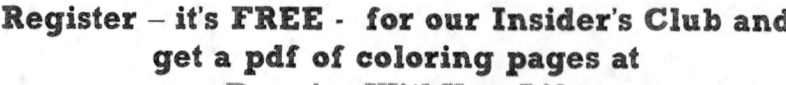

ISBN: 978-0-9944230-4-7

Published by Seshat Publications
13/56 Carl Street, Woolloongabba Qld 4102 Australia
Web: www.SeshatPublications.com
Email: Support@SeshatPublishing.com

Printed by CreateSpace

Compilation and design by Richard Wineberg
Email: rkw@RichardWineberg.com

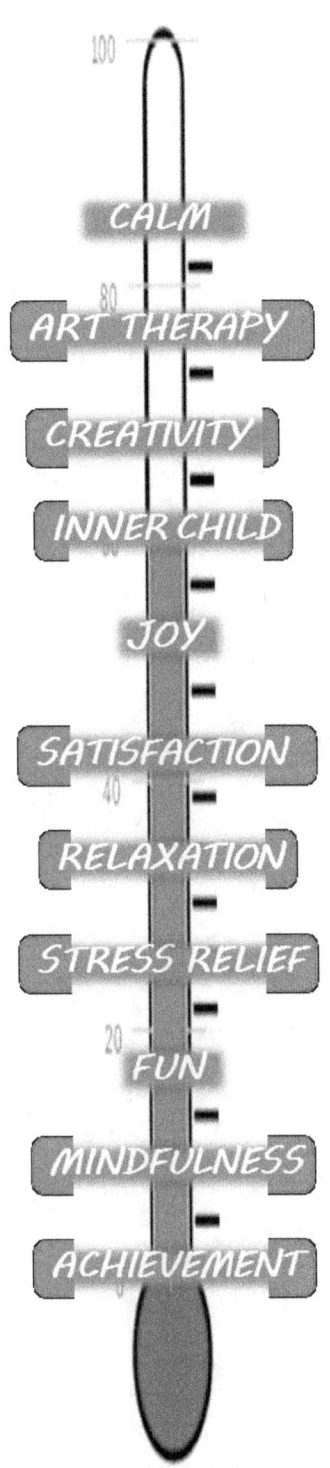

Getting started...

Each page is printed only on the right hand side. It helps stop bleeding or hand pressure affecting the next drawing.

Colored pencils and crayons are fine to use.

If you are planning to use wet markers, pens or watercolor paint, please place a sheet of paper or cardboard under your current page. It's also a good idea to avoid excessive wetness.

Start on any page you like. There's no fixed order.

Enjoying the process...

Just relax and have fun with the coloring process.

It's OK to:
- ✓ Add your own creative lines or drawings.
- ✓ Add color outside lines for effect.
- ✓ Leave areas uncolored for creative effect.

Sharing this coloring book...

Sharing with your spouse, partner, grandchildren or children enhances the creative experience and relationship for you both.

Artists and Writers ...

Often lose track of time and awareness outside of their work. If you should encounter this sensation take notice of how calm and unstressed you are. Acknowledge the joy, the creativity being experienced and keep coloring.

**Change is not a four letter word...
but often your reaction to it is!**

Jeffrey Gitomer

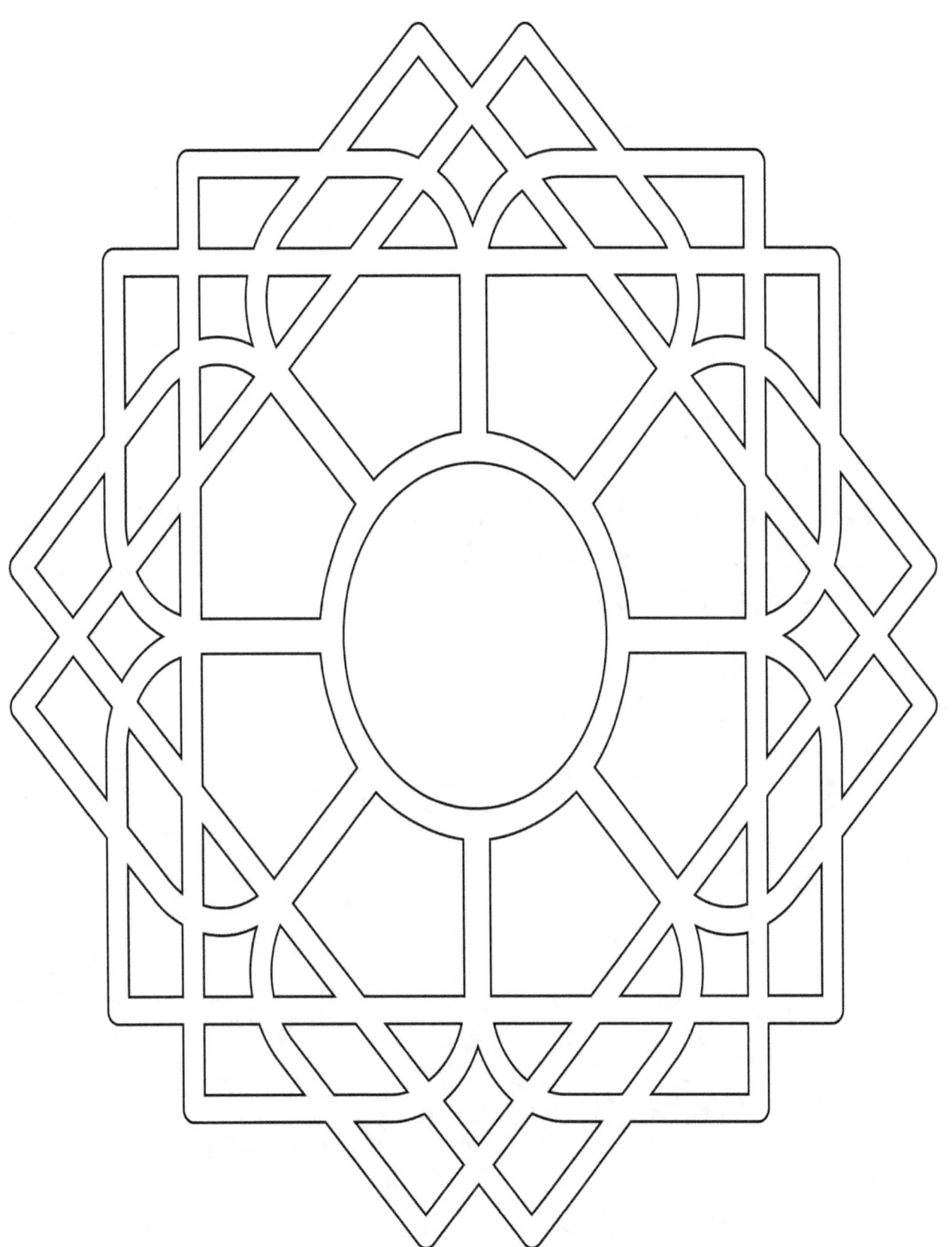

Opportunity is missed by most people because it is dressed in overalls and looks like work.

Thomas Eddison

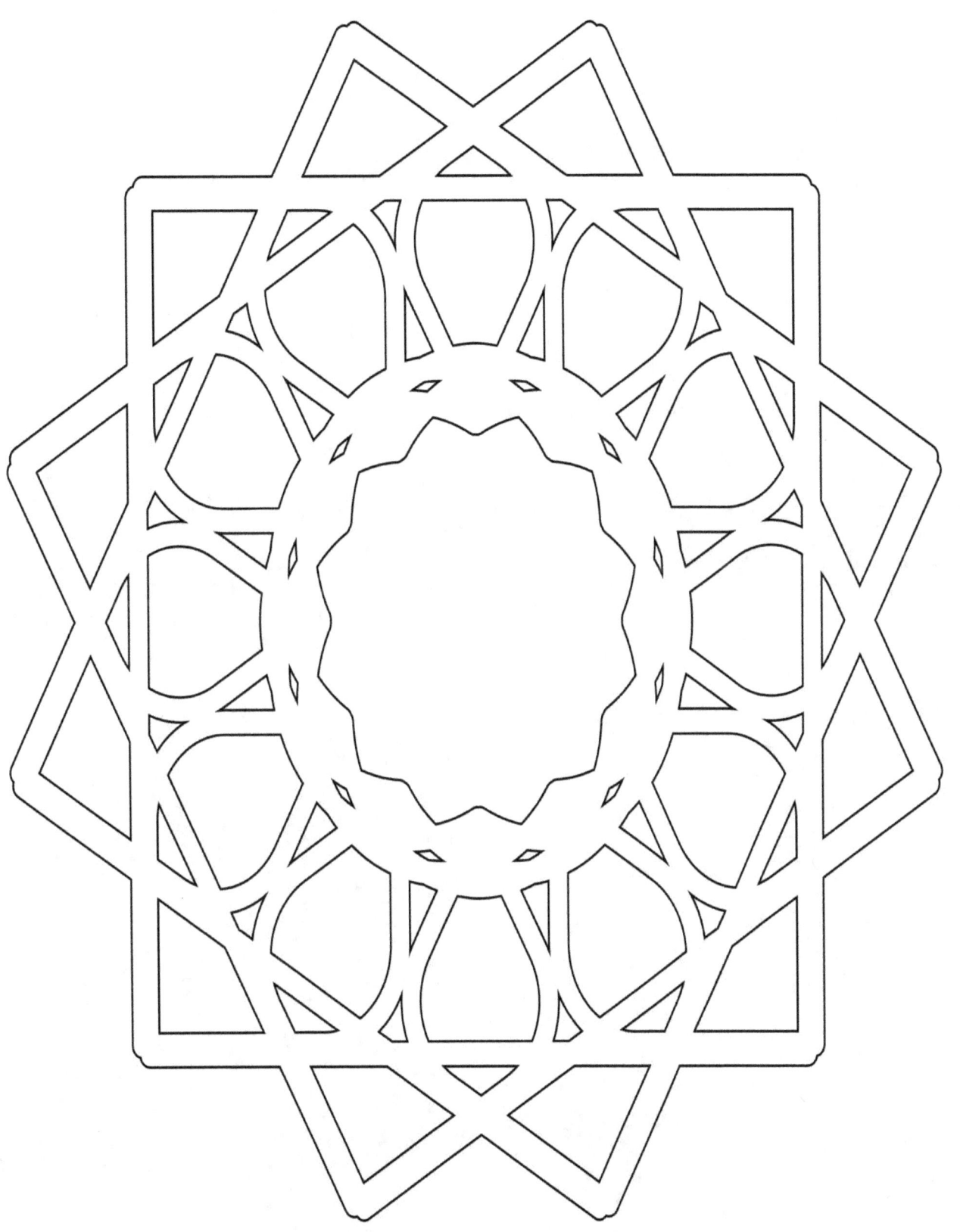

A day without sunshine is like, you know, night.

Steve Martin

If you try to fail, and succeed, which have you done?

George Carlin

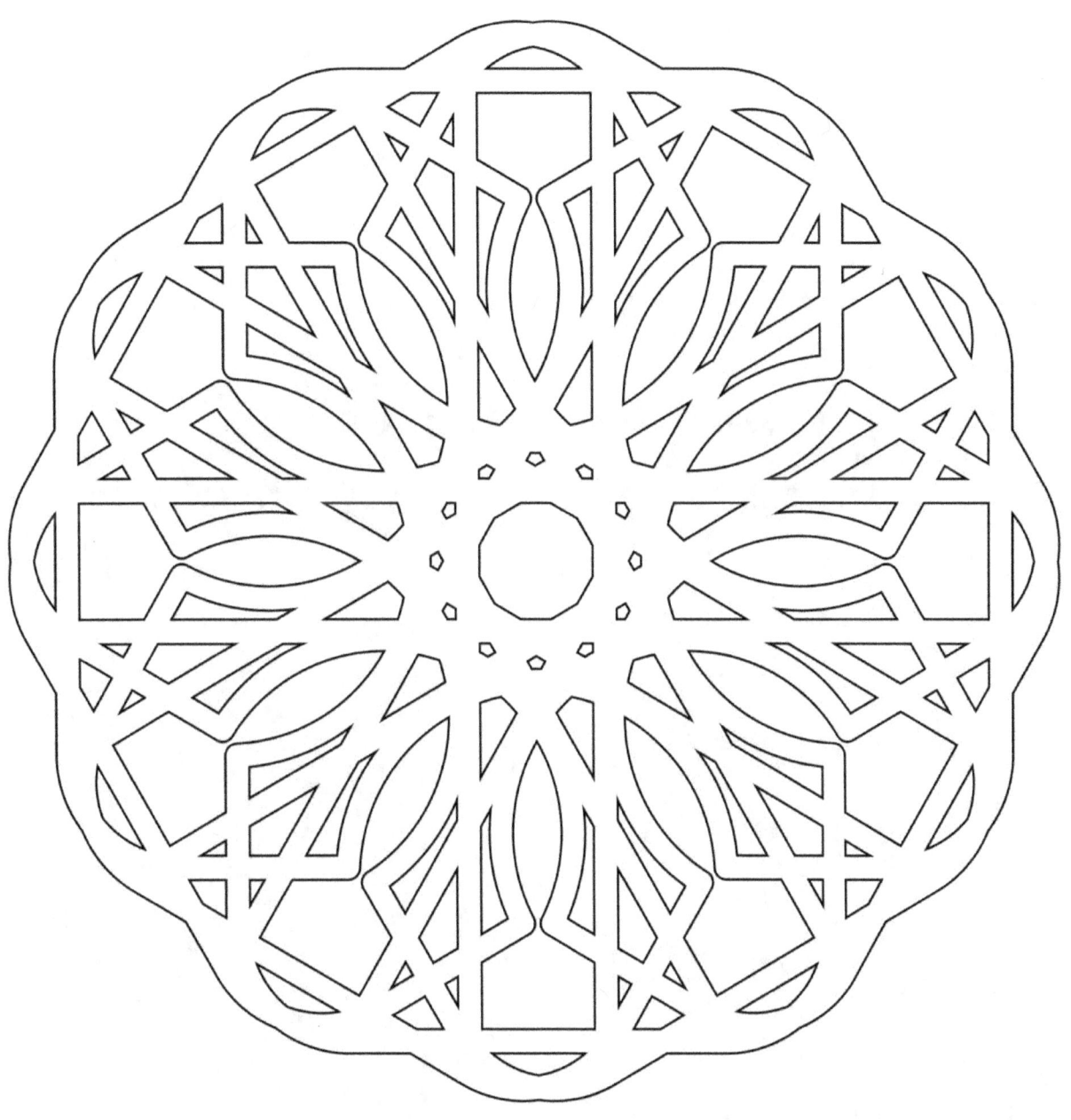

**You can't wait for inspiration.
You have to go after it with a club.**

Jack London

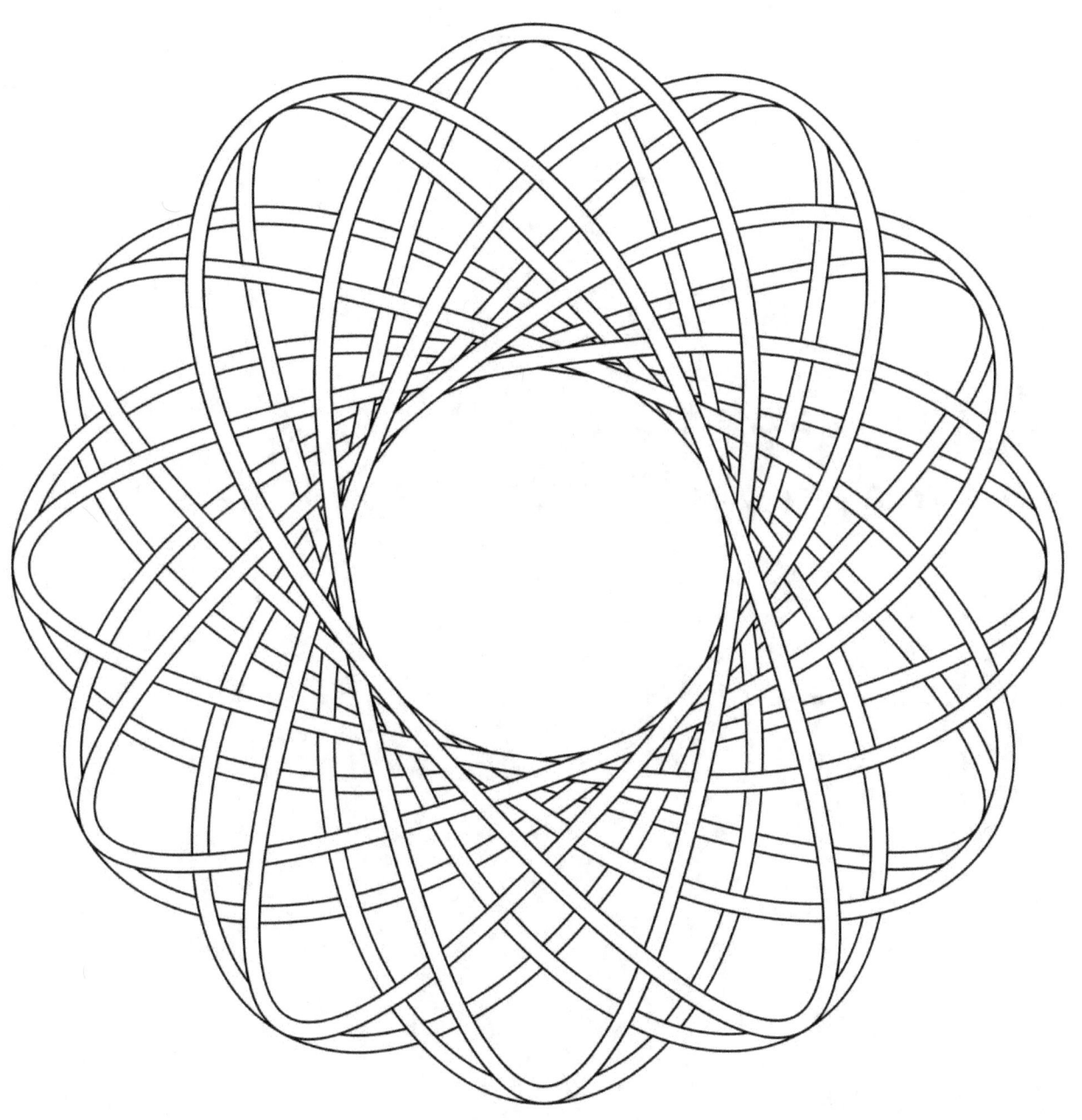

If you're going to be thinking, you may as well think big.

Donald Trump

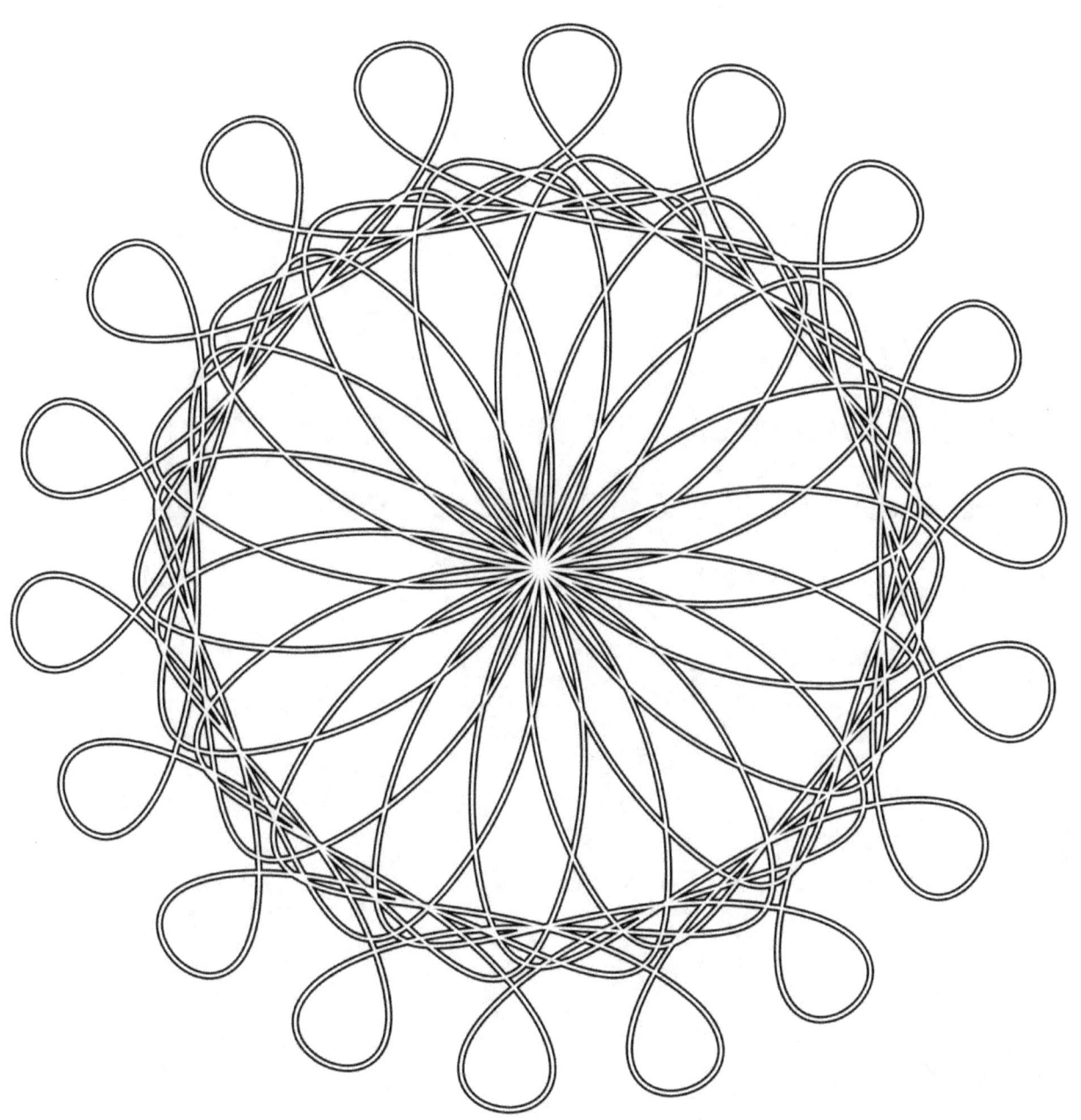

Opportunity does not knock, it presents itself when you beat down the door.

Kyle Chandler

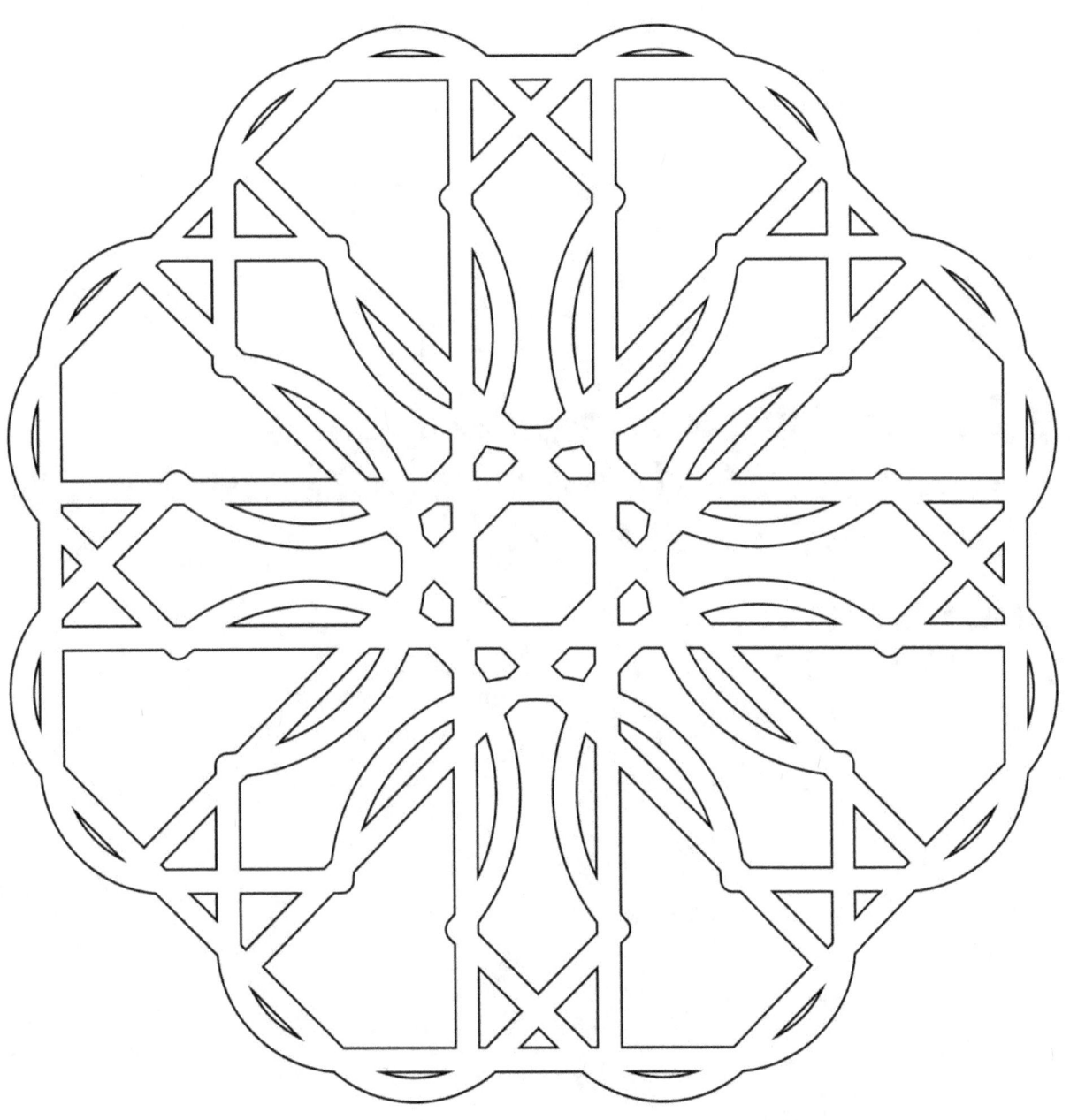

Great spirits have always encountered violent opposition from mediocre minds.

Albert Einstein

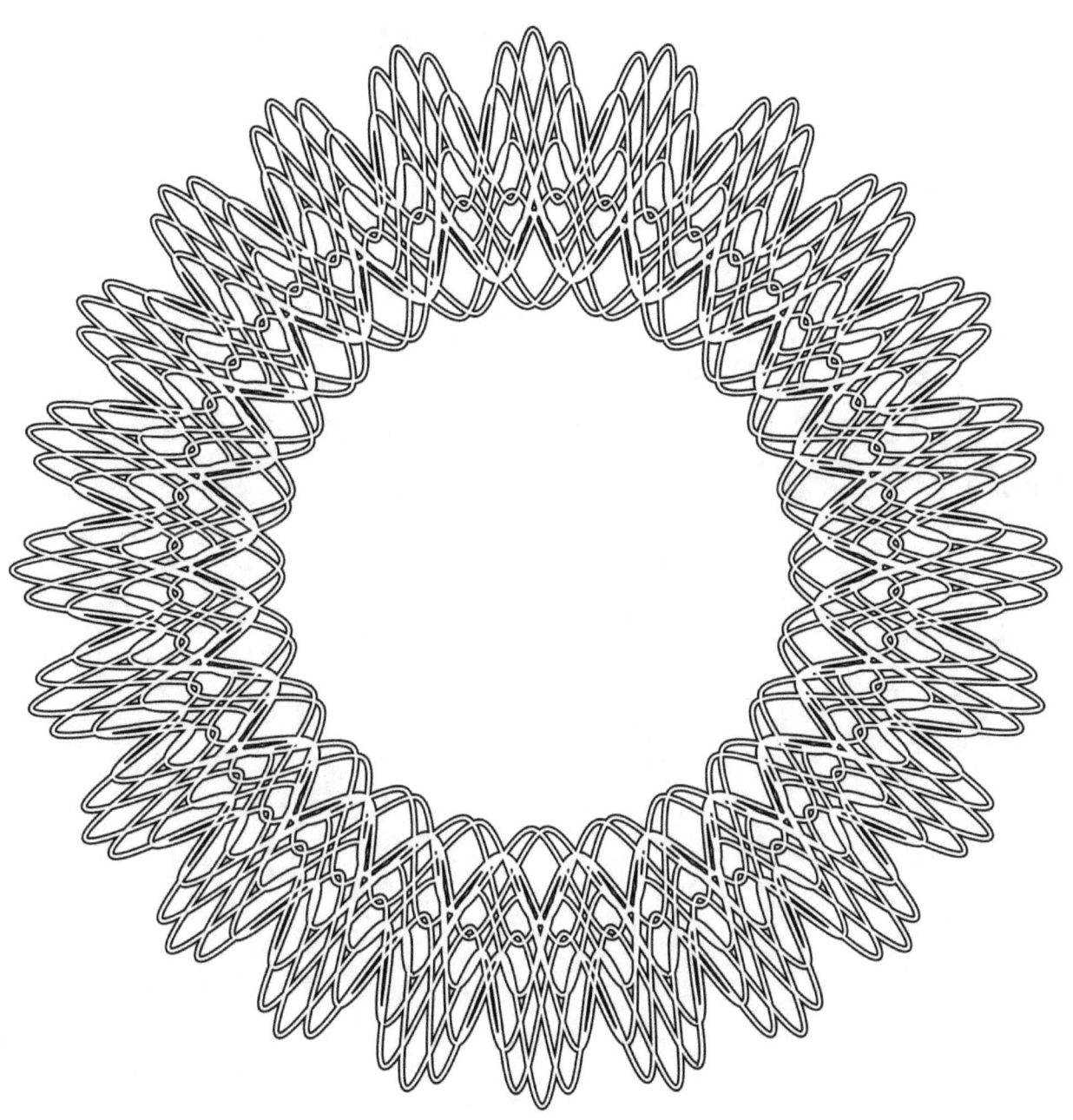

People say nothing is impossible, but I do nothing every day.

A.A. Milne

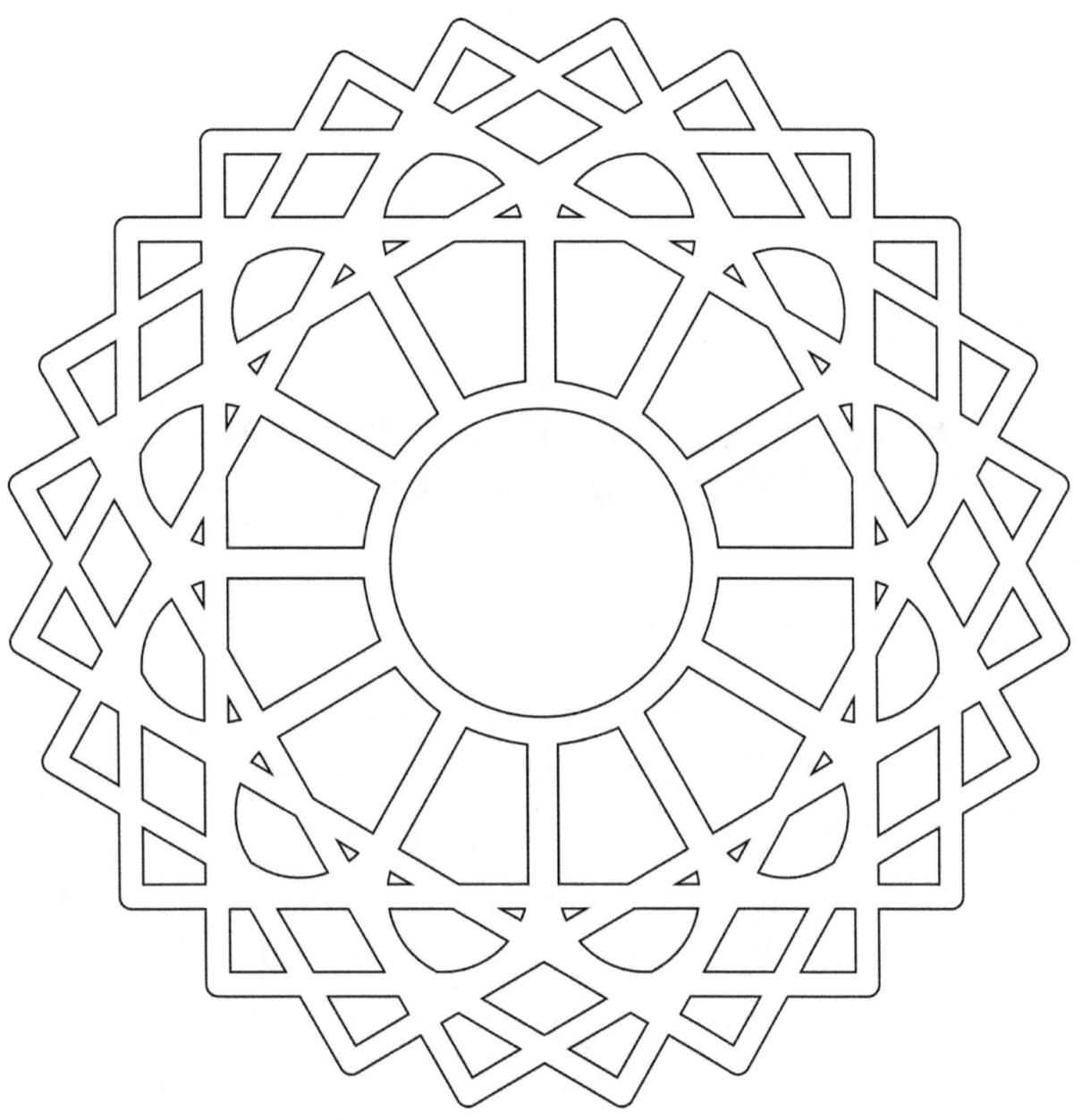

A diamond is merely a lump of coal that did well under pressure.

Unknown

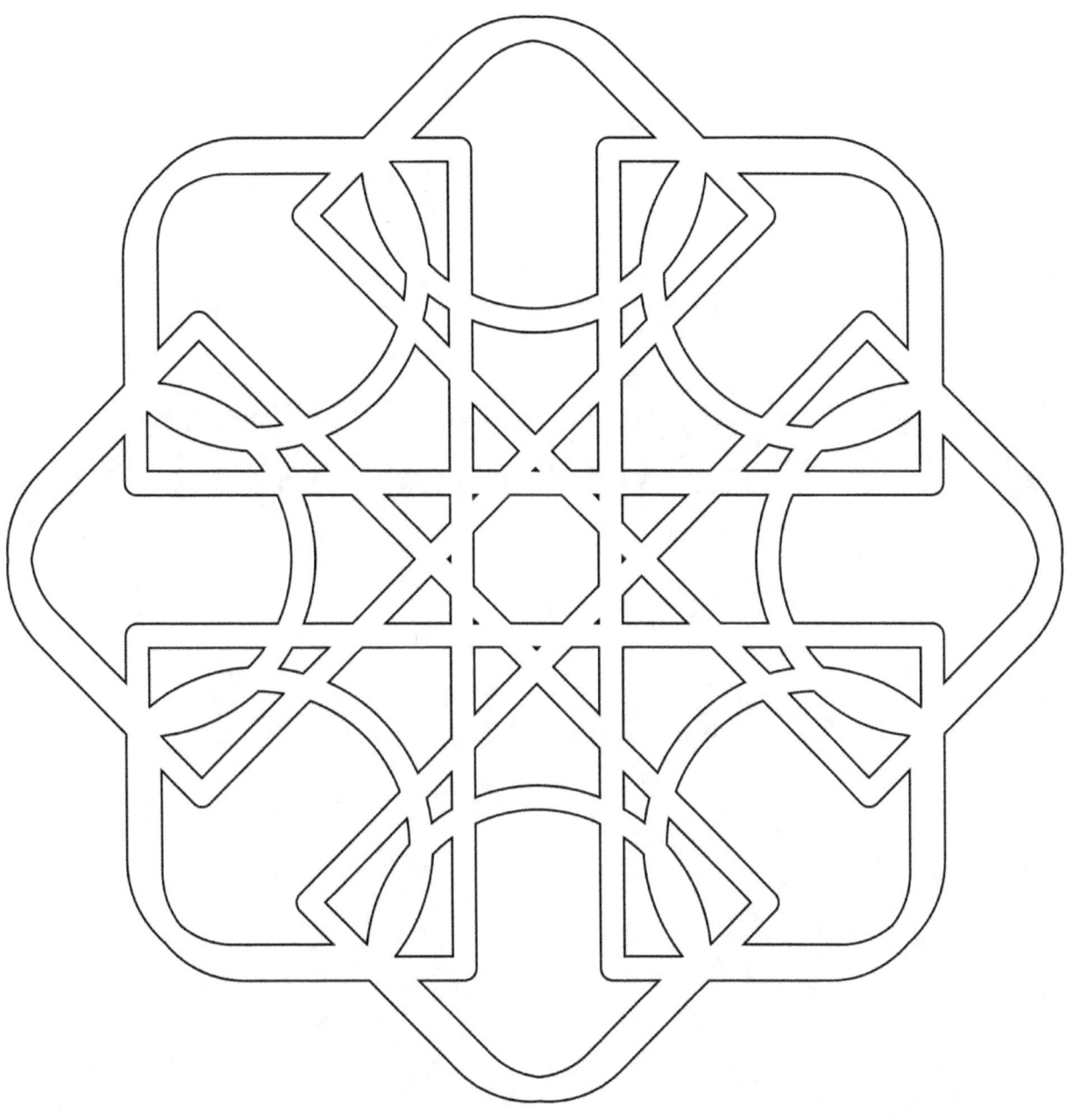

Even if you are on the right track, you'll get run over if you just sit there.

Will Rogers

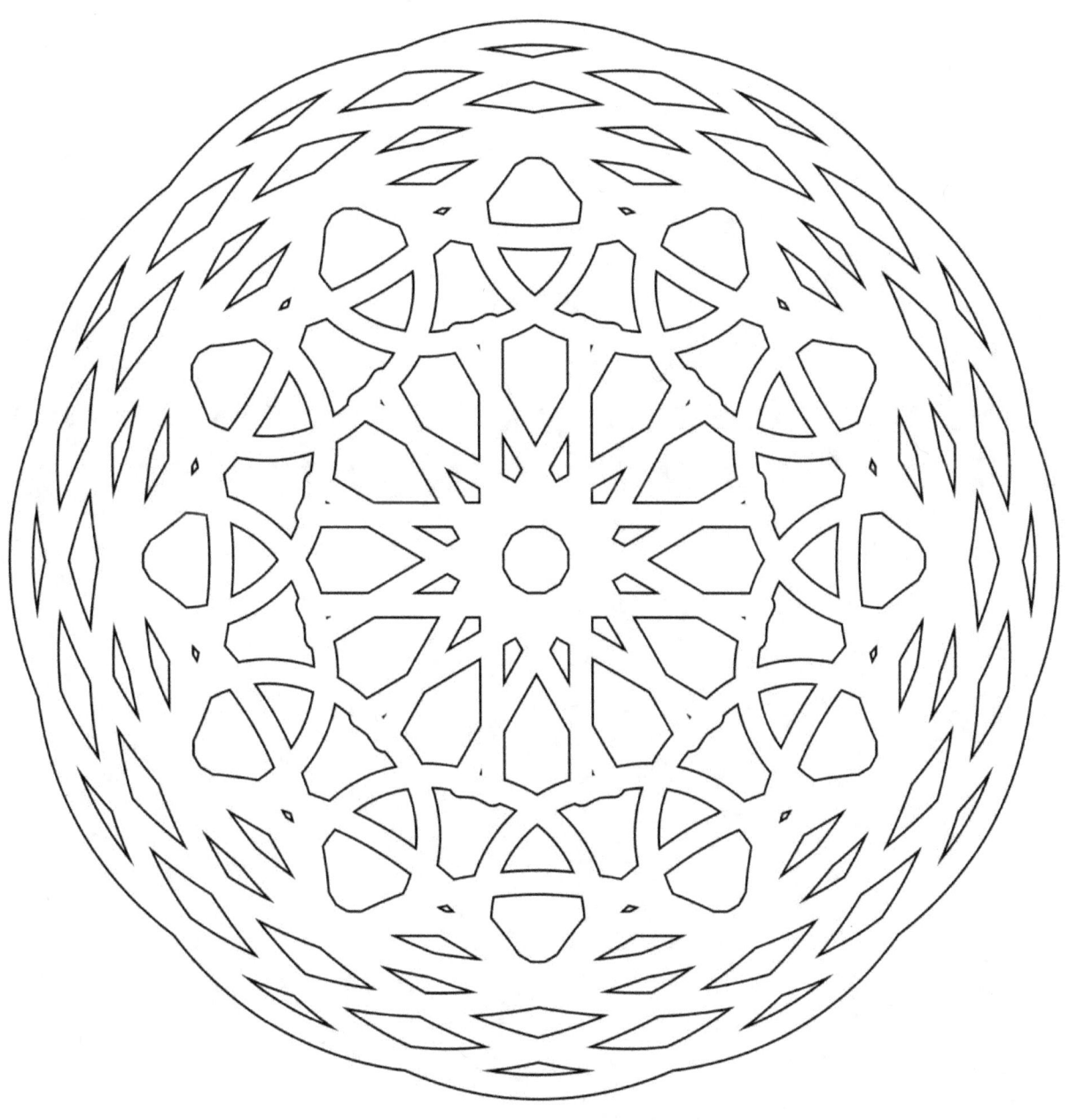

Never put off until tomorrow what you can do the day after tomorrow.

Mark Twain

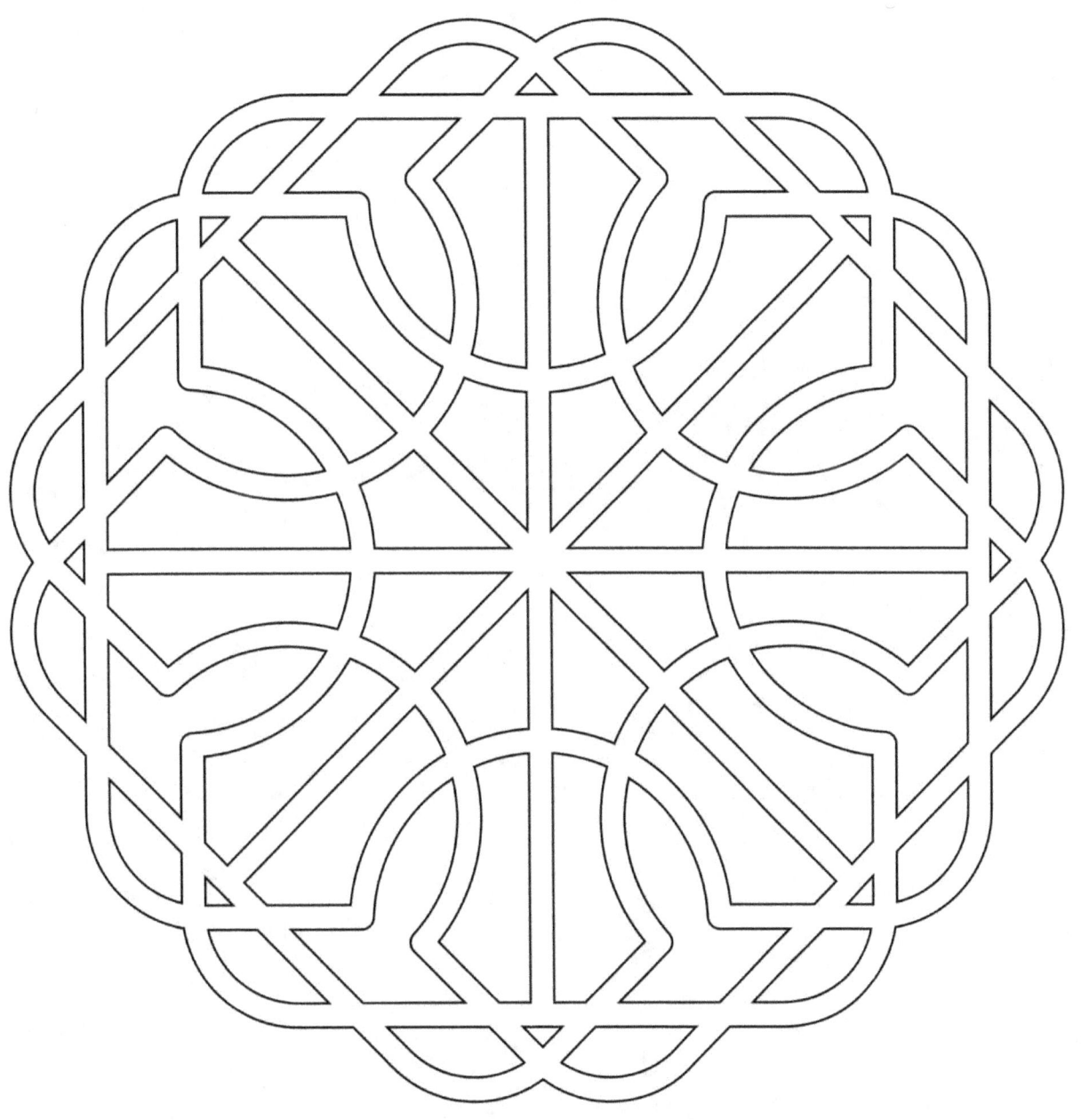

**Try to be like the turtle –
at ease in your own shell.**

Bill Copeland

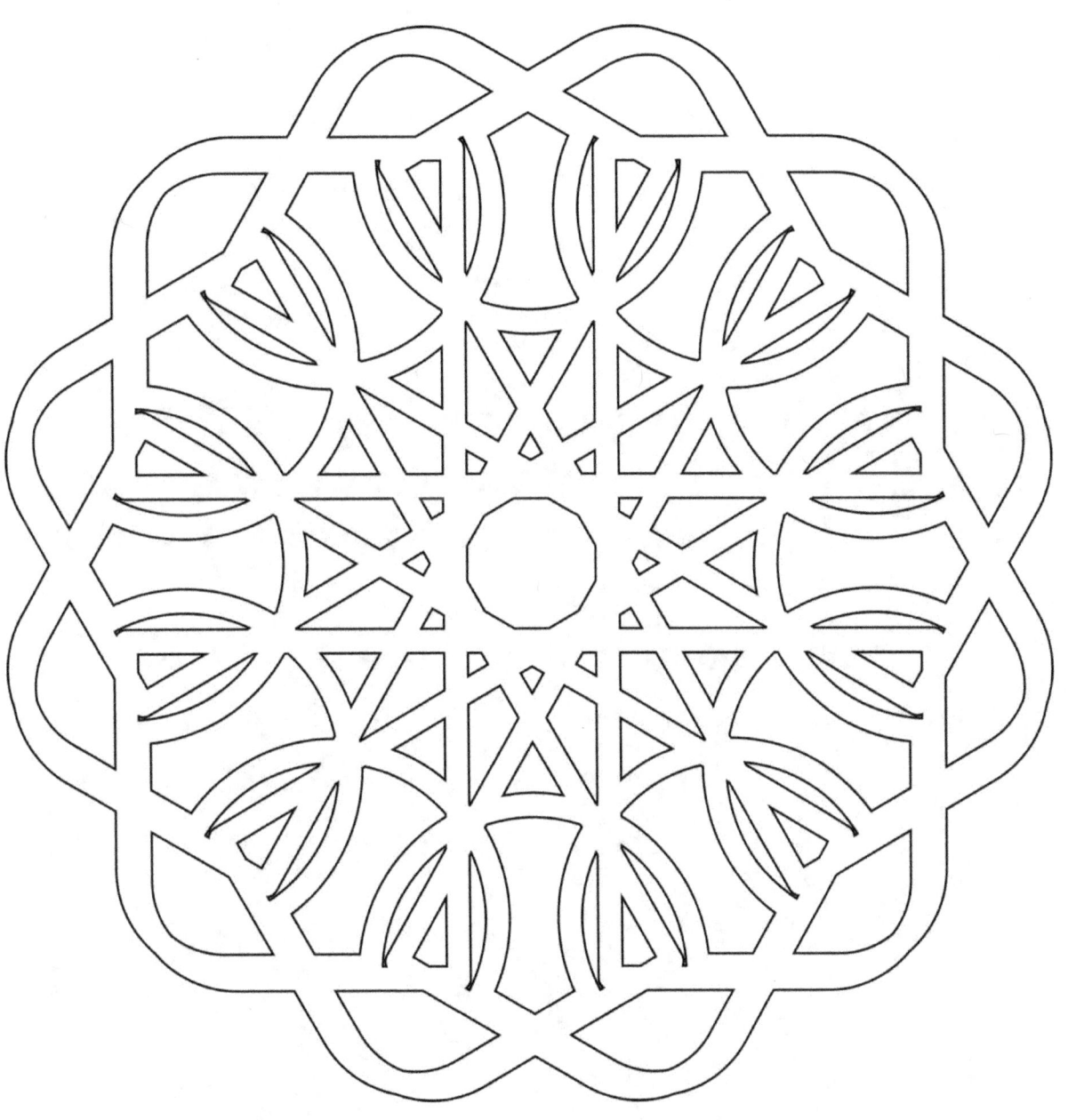

Follow your passion, stay true to yourself, never follow someone else's path unless you're in the woods and you're lost and you see a path then by all means you should follow that.

Ellen Degeneres

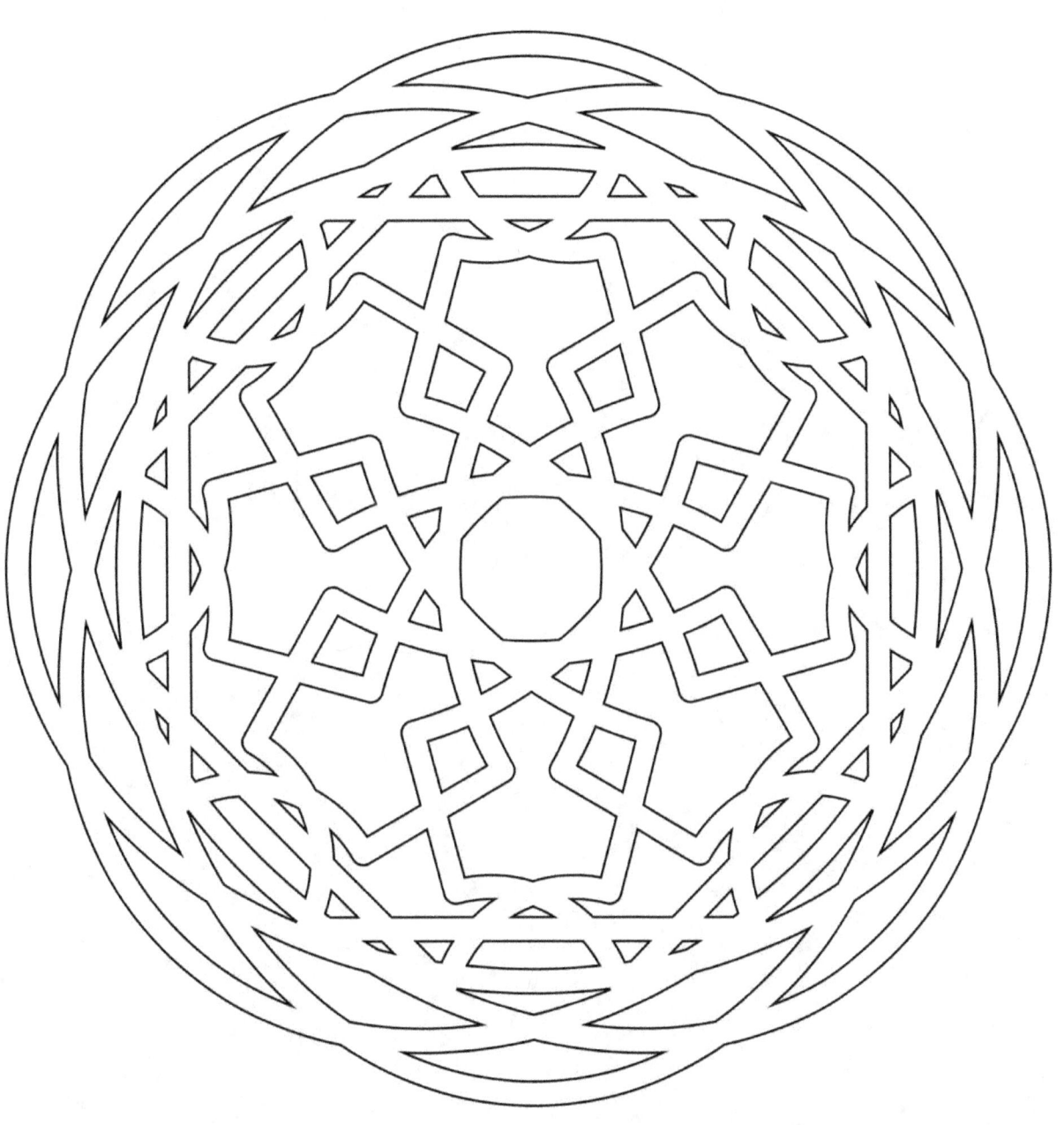

Life is like a sewer...

what you get out of it depends on what you put into it.

Tom Lehrer

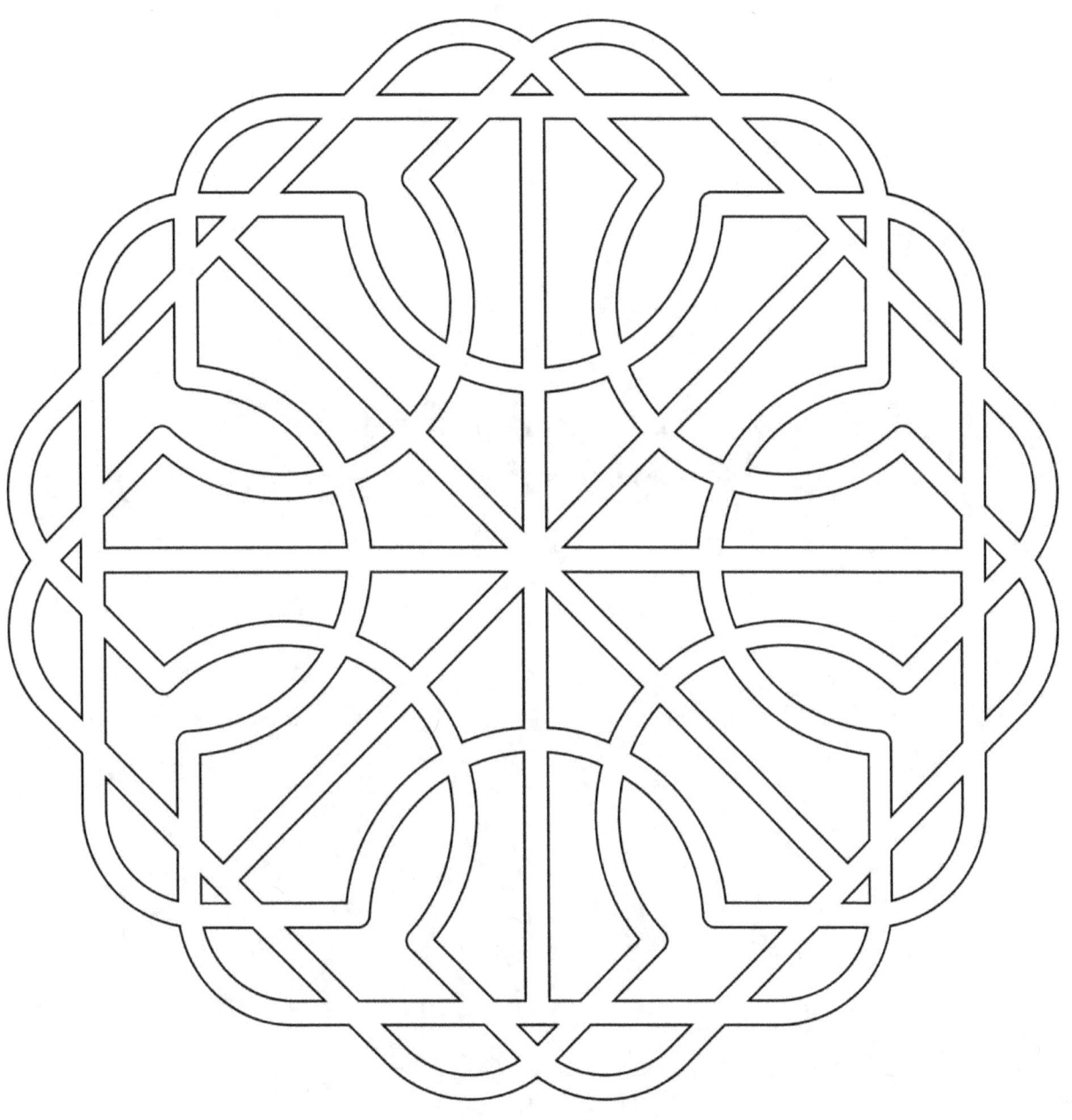

Never let your sense of morals prevent you from doing what is right.

Isaac Asimov

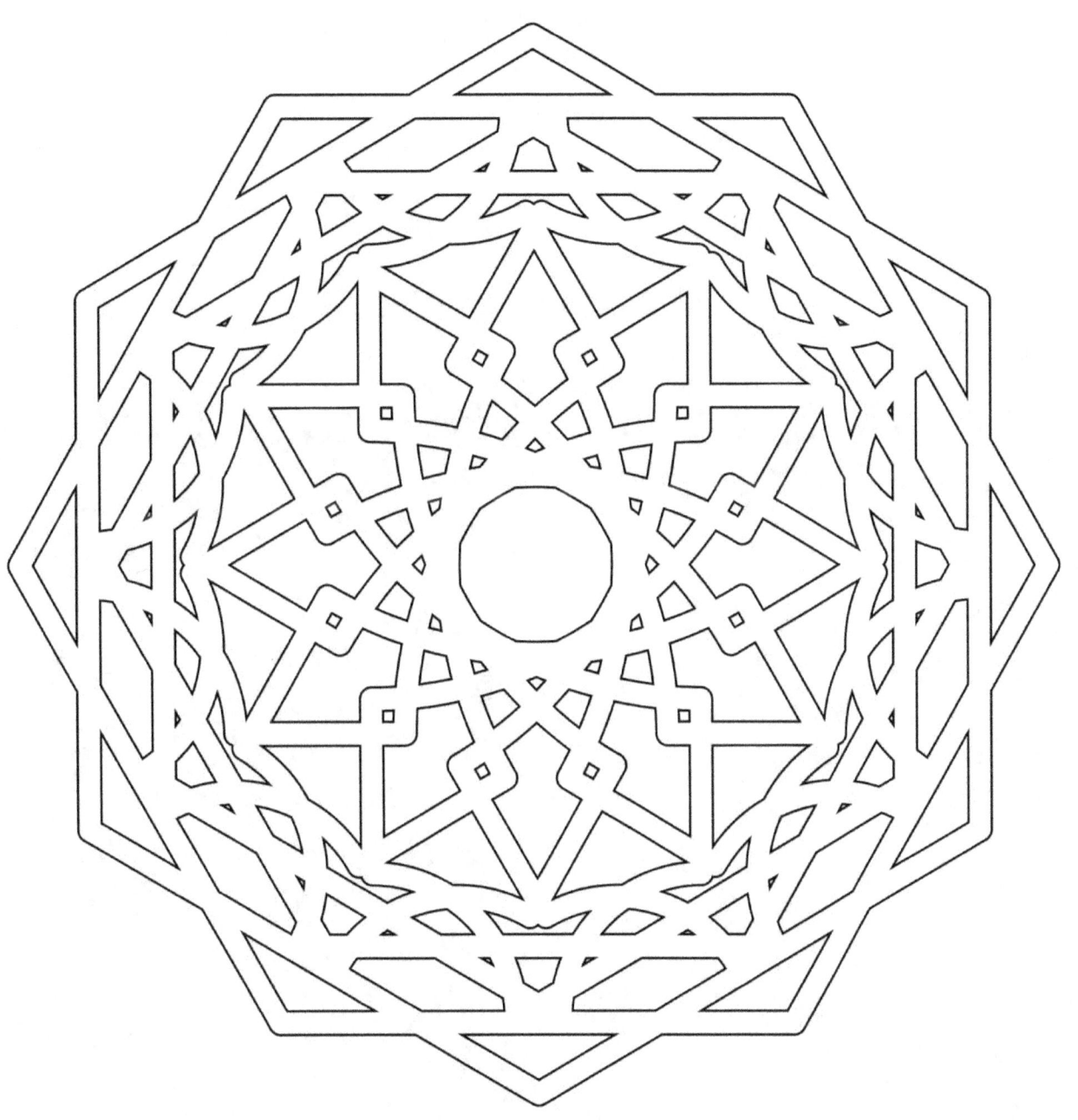

Failure is the condiment that gives success its flavor.

Truman Capote

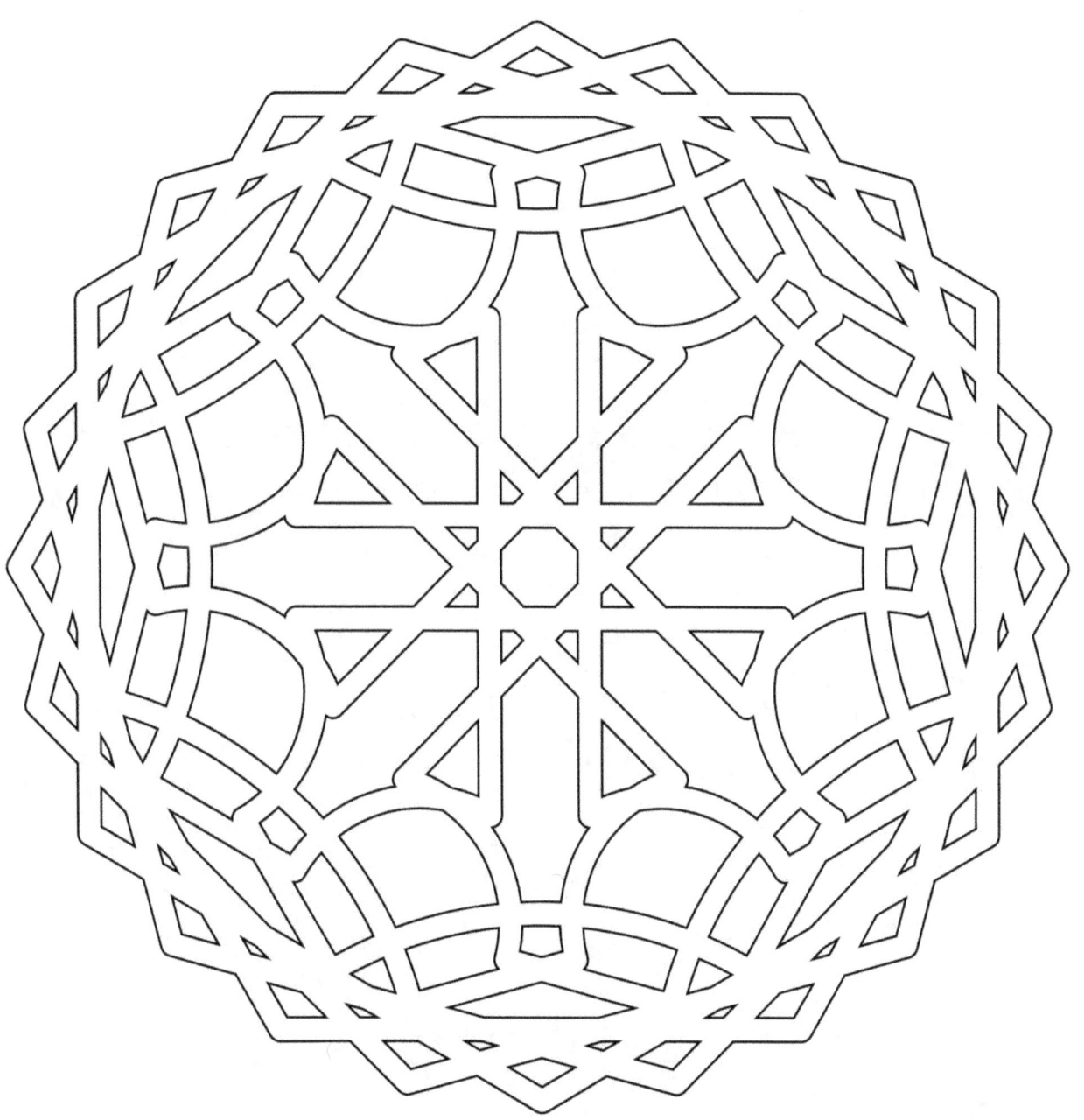

**People often say that motivation doesn't last.
Well, neither does bathing –
that's why we recommend it daily.**

Zig Ziglar

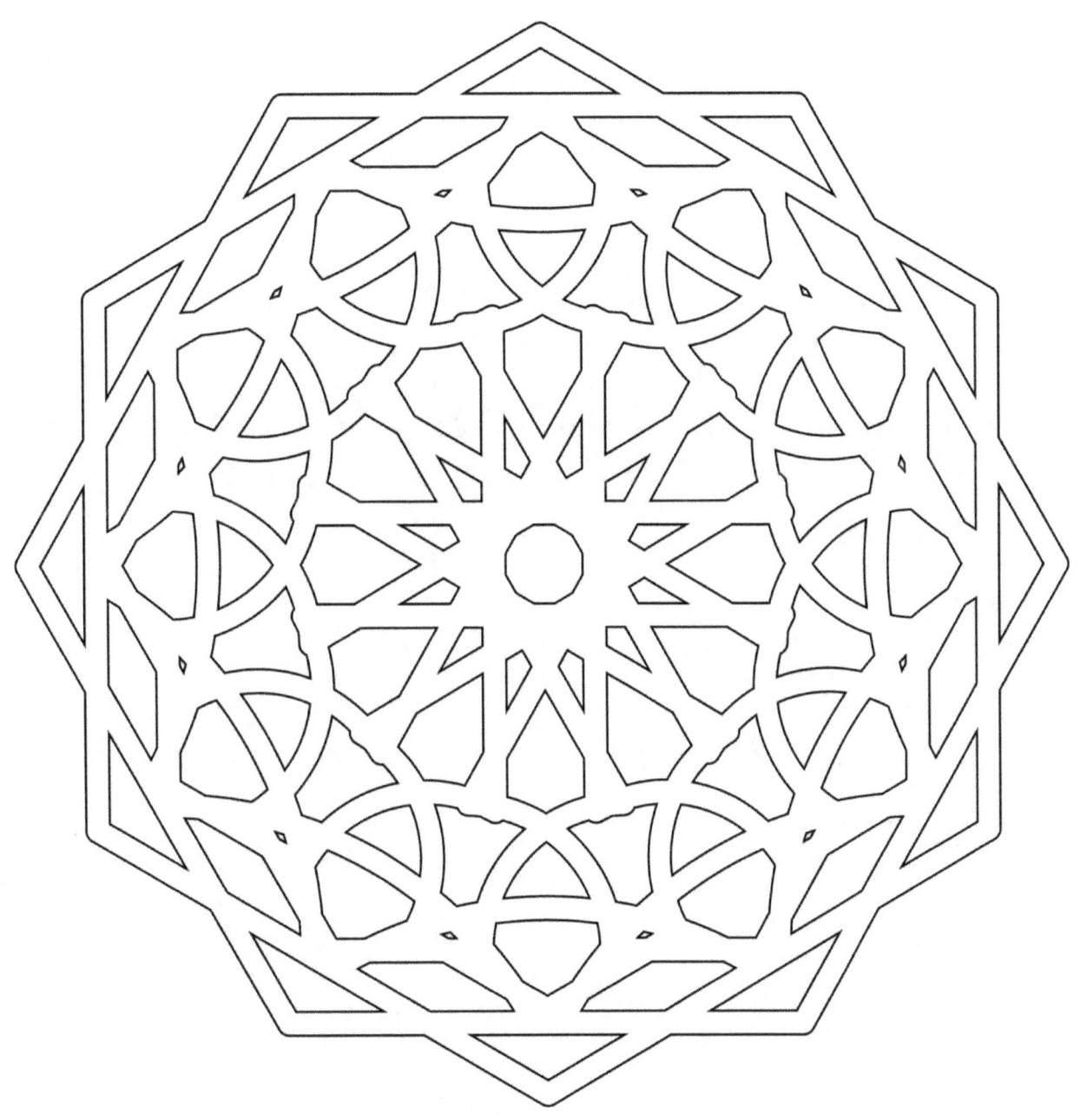

If you think you are too small to make a difference, try sleeping with a mosquito.

Dalai Lama

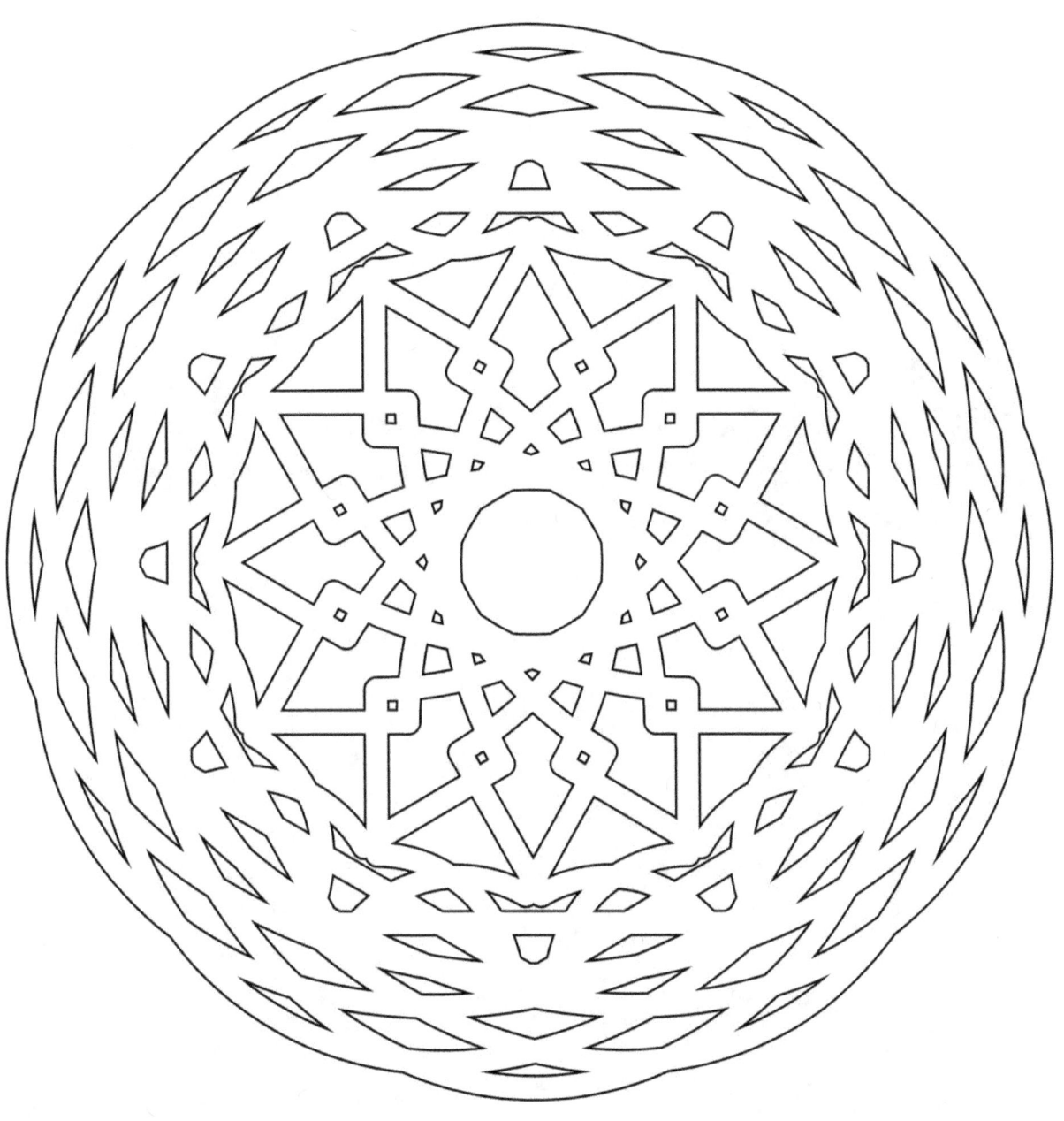

When I hear somebody sigh, 'Life is hard,' I am always tempted to ask, 'Compared to what?'

Sydney Harris

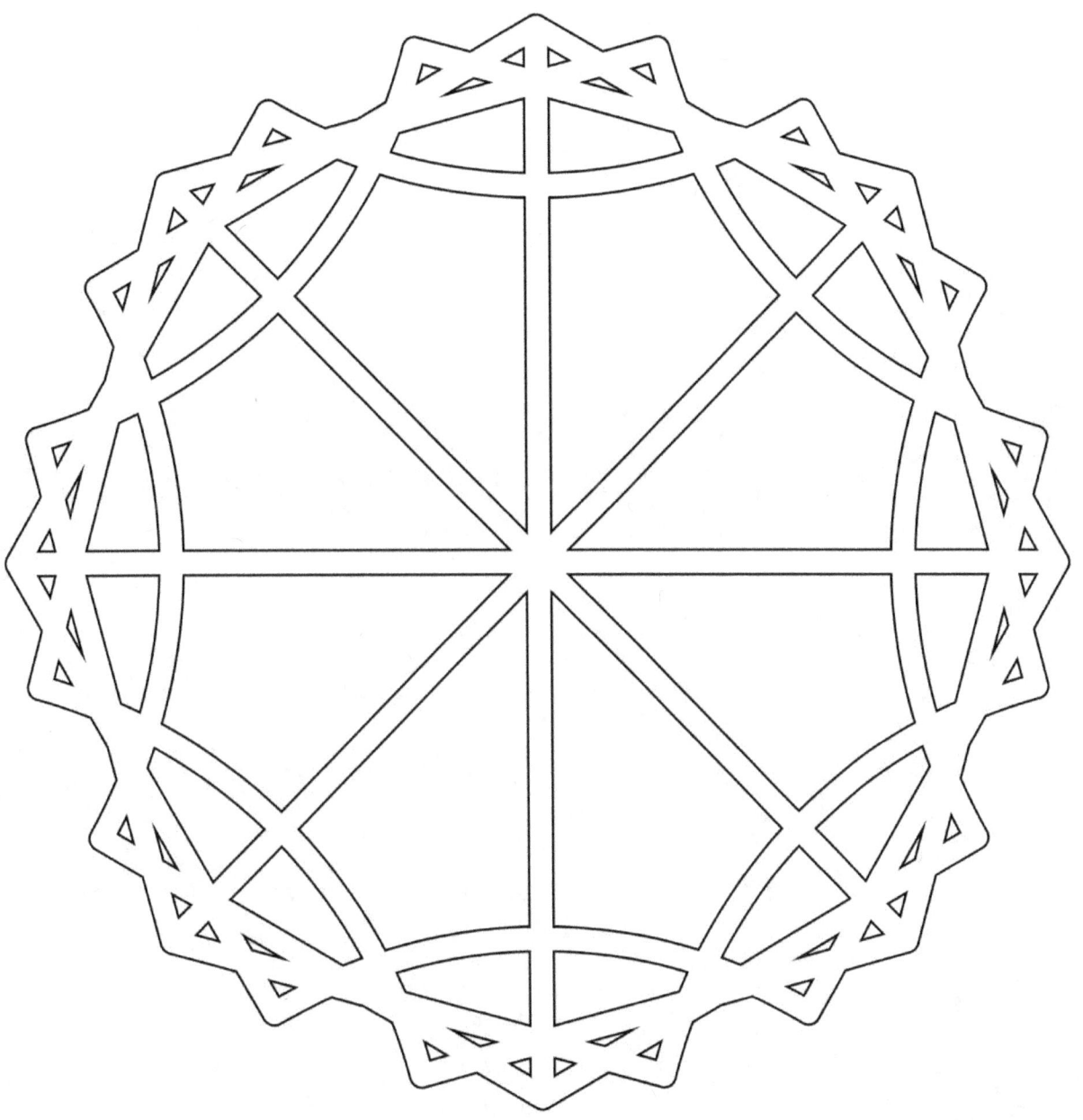

I always wanted to be somebody, but now I realize I should have been more specific.

Lily Tomlin

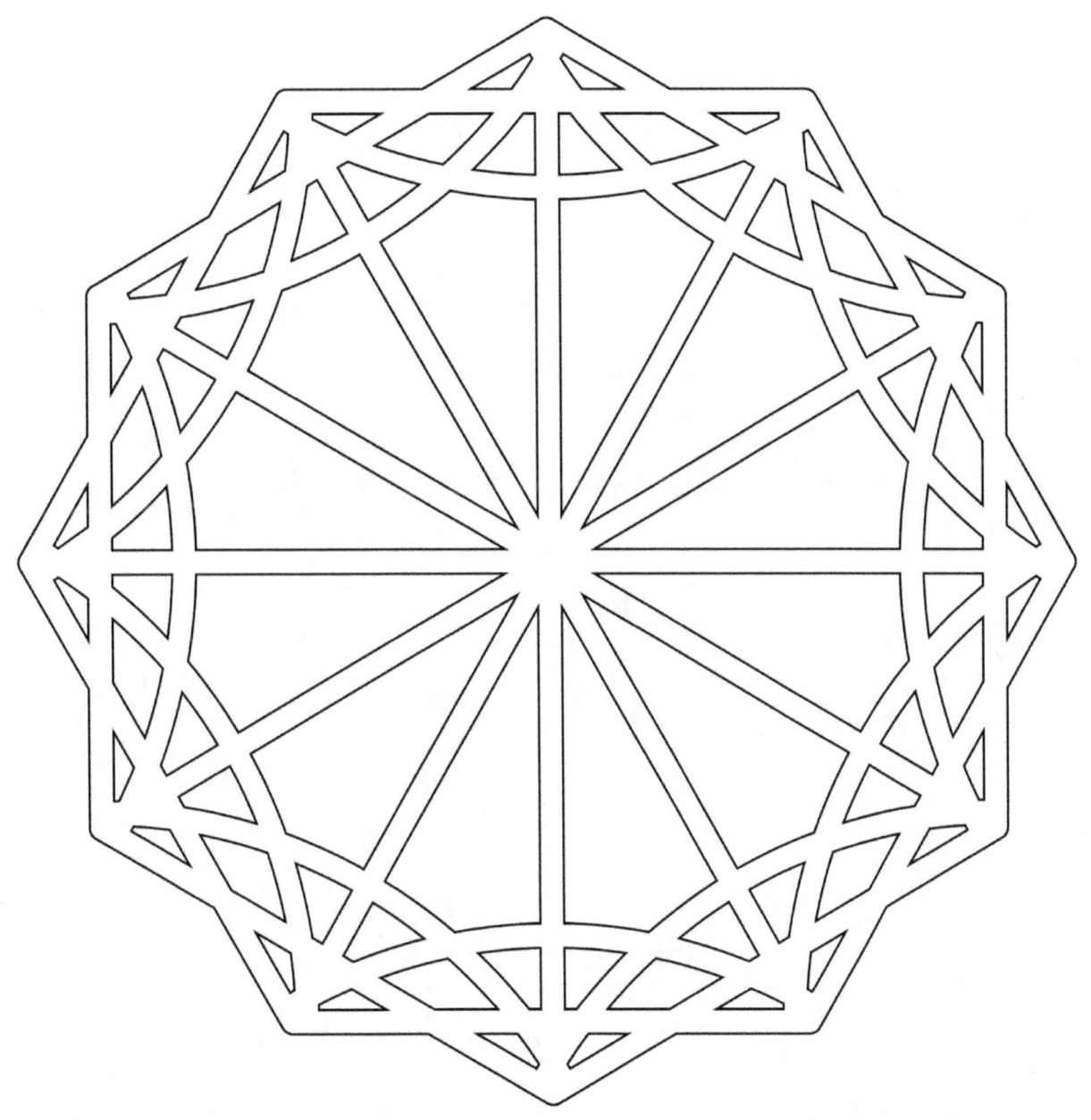

Well-behaved women seldom make history.

Laurel Thatcher Ulrich

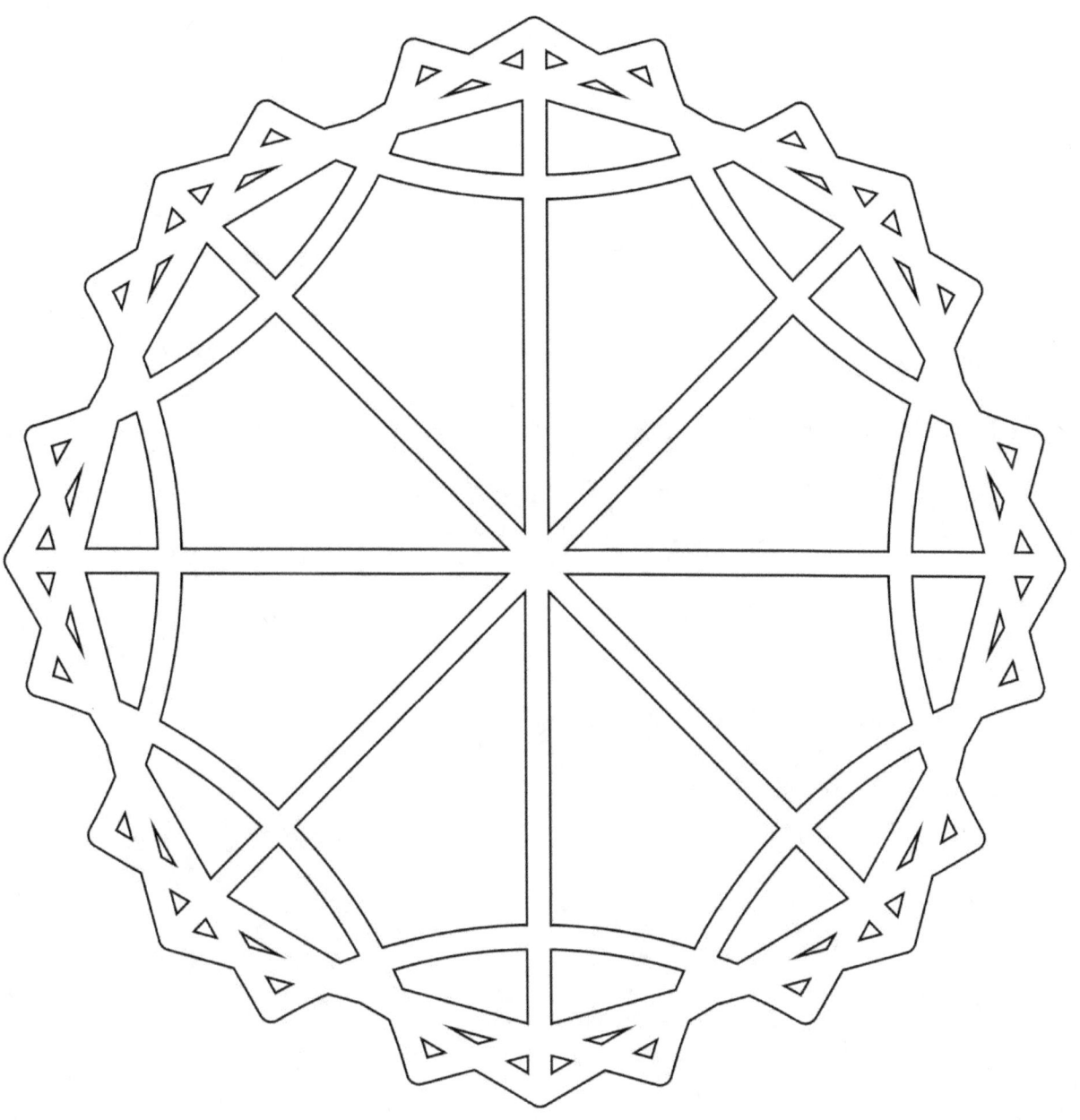

If you're going to be able to look back on something and laugh about it, you might as well laugh about it now.

Marie Osmond

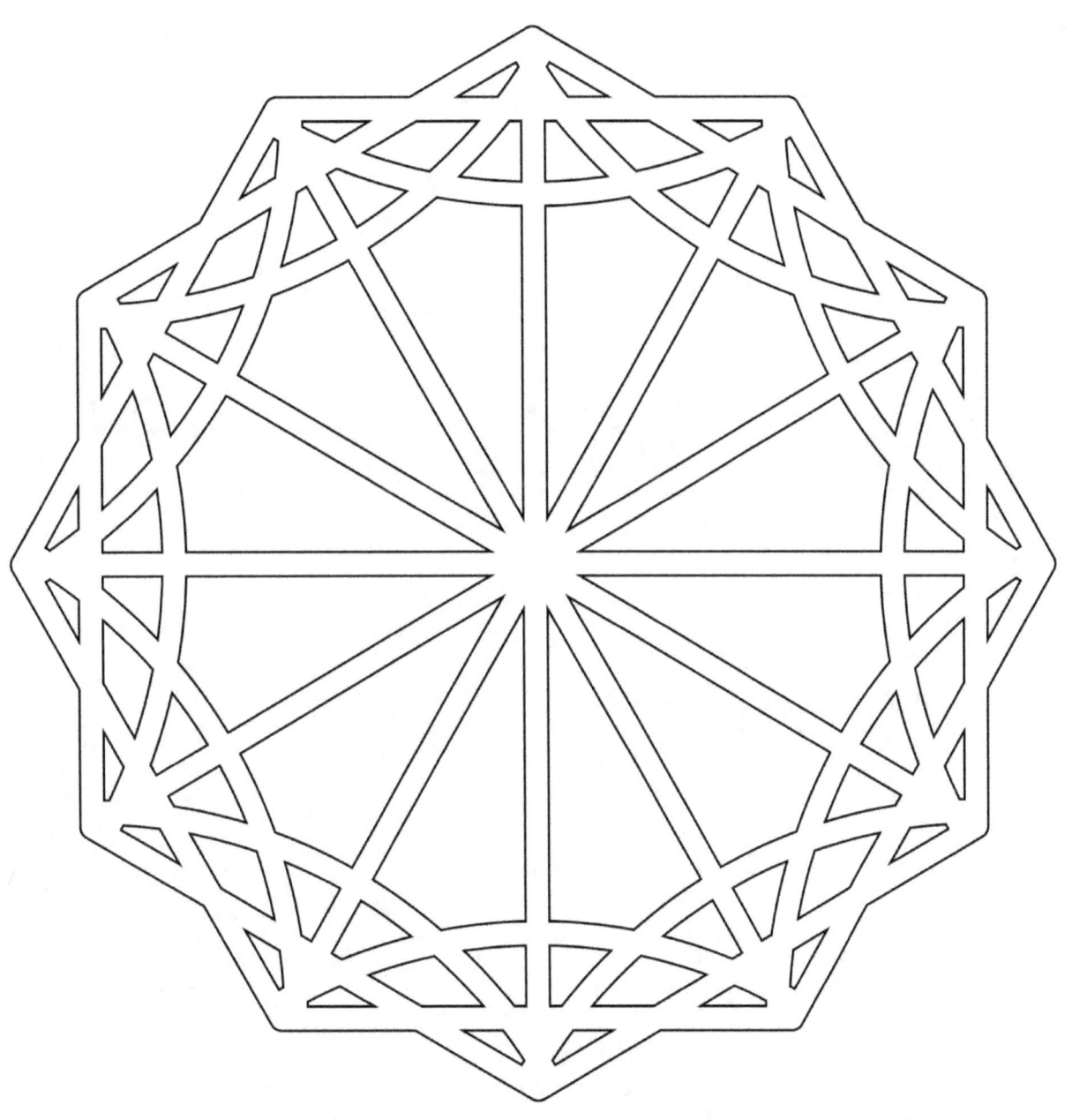

There are no traffic jams along the extra mile.

Roger Staubach

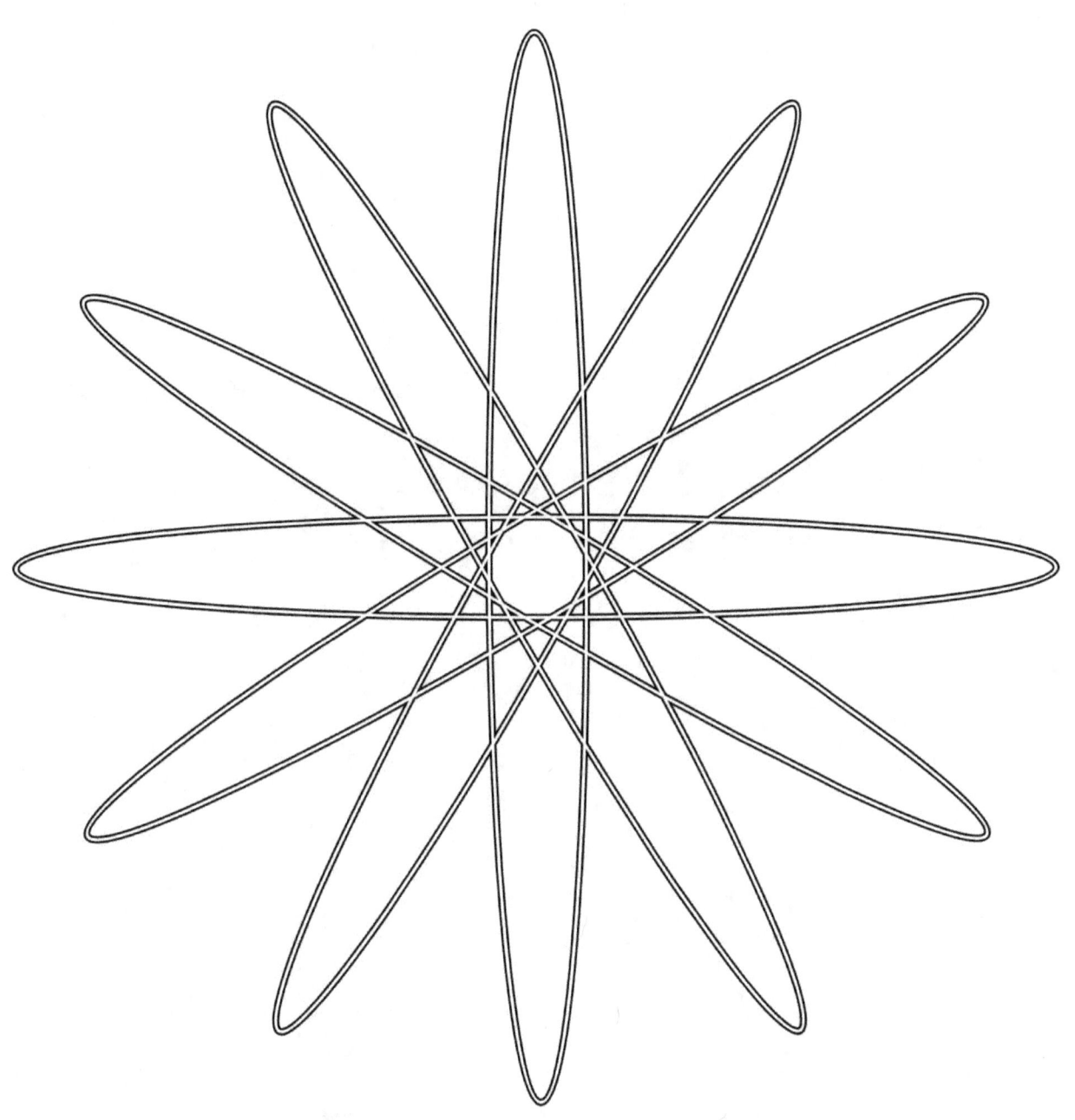

**Life is like photography.
You need the negatives to develop.**
Unknown

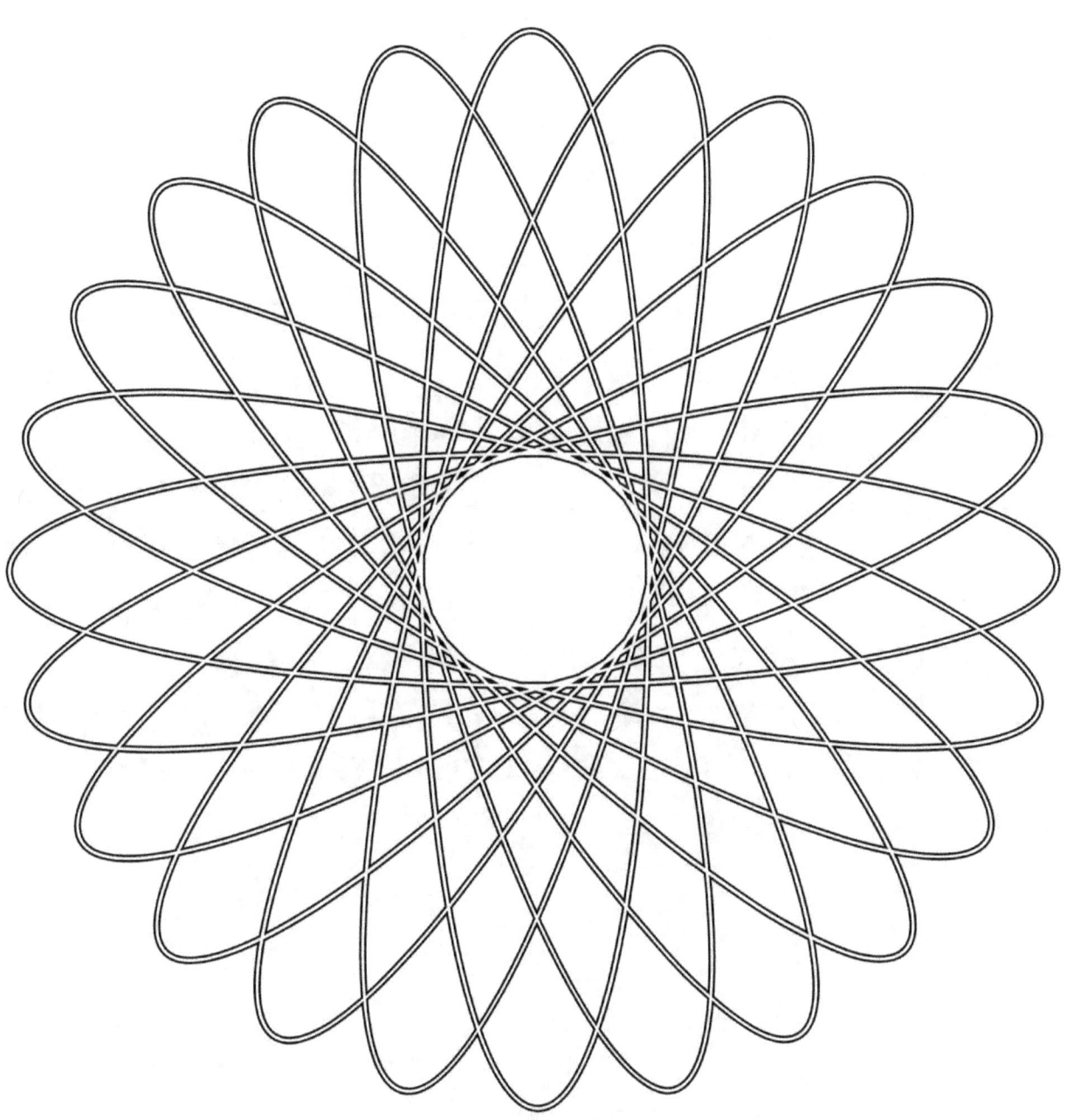

I'm bored' is a useless thing to say. I mean, you live in a great, big, vast world that you've seen none percent of. Even the inside of your own mind is endless; it goes on forever, inwardly, do you understand? The fact that you're alive is amazing, so you don't get to say 'I'm bored. –

Louis C.K.

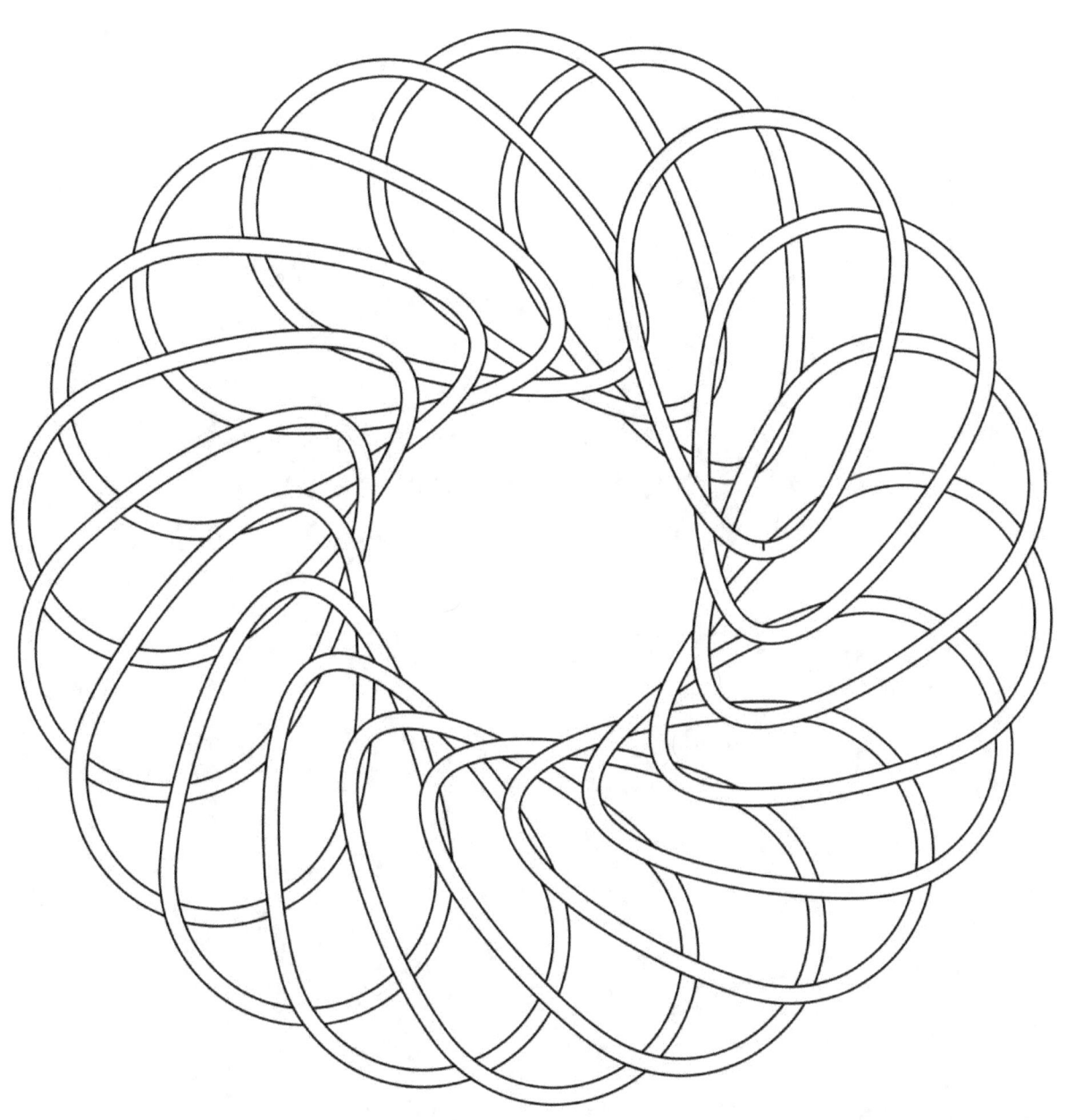

Life is a blank canvass, and you need to throw all the paint on it you can.
Danny Kaye

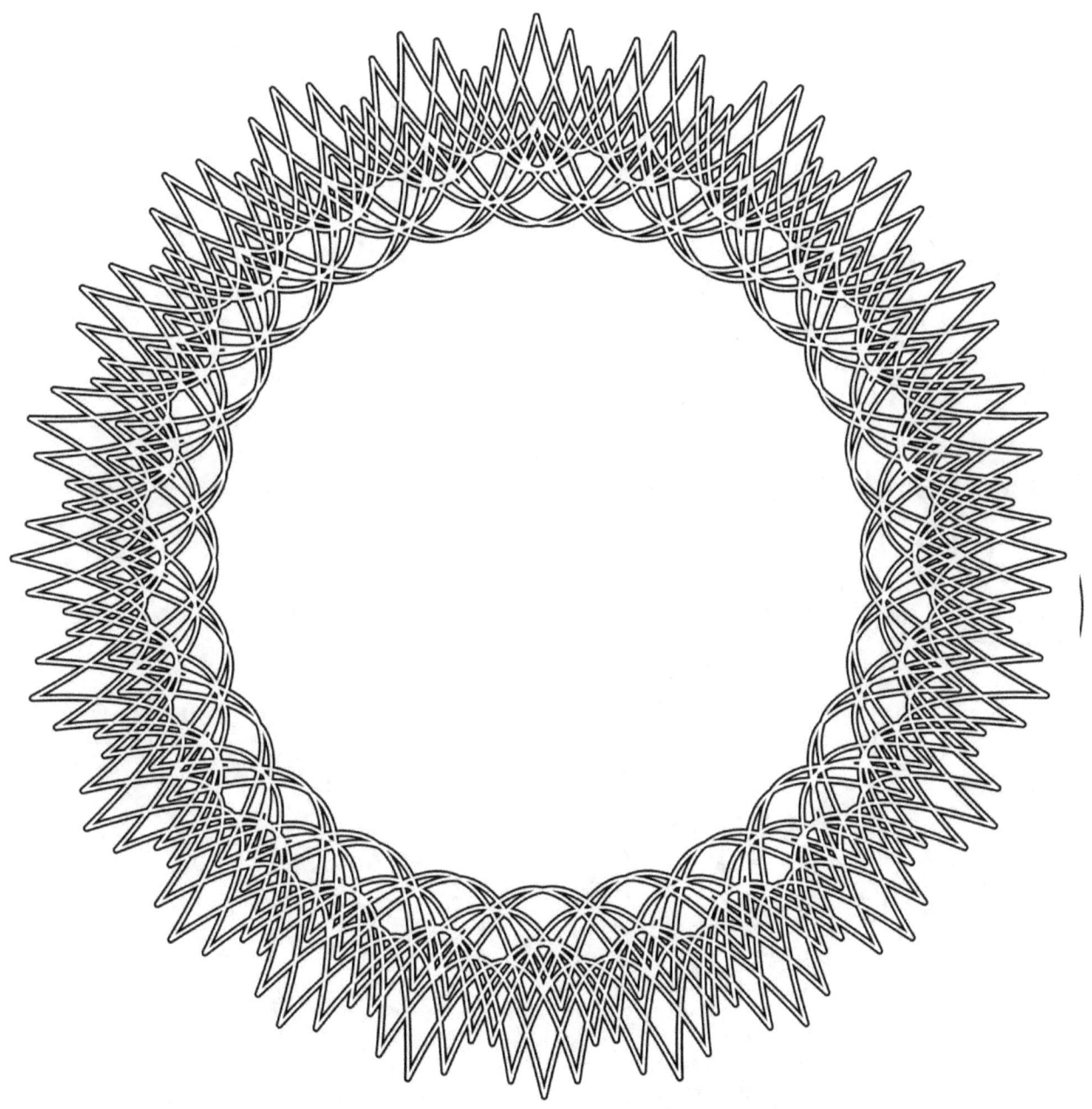

If you hit the target every time it's too near or too big.

Tom Hirshfield

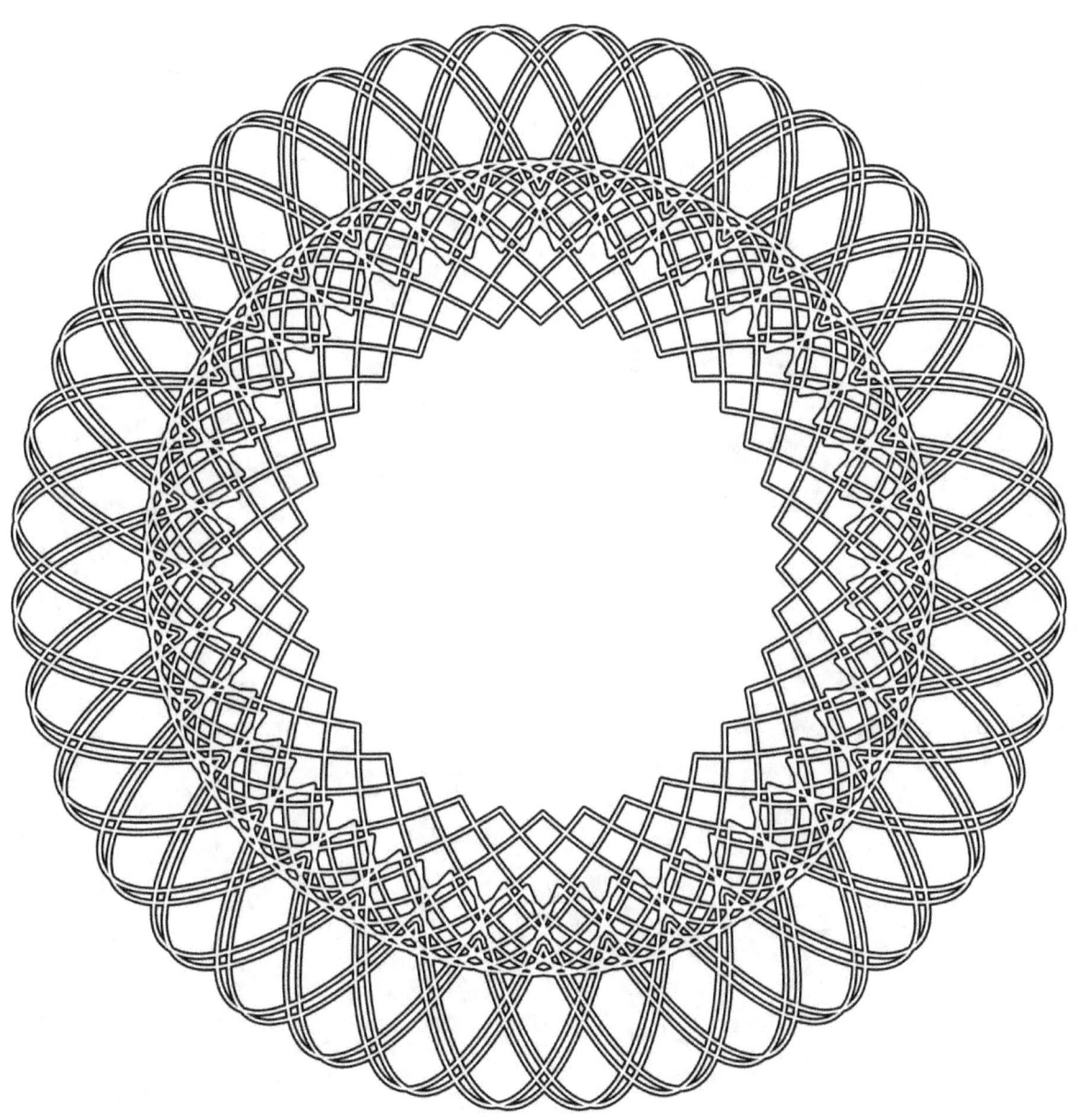

There's never enough time to do all the nothing you want.

Bill Watterson

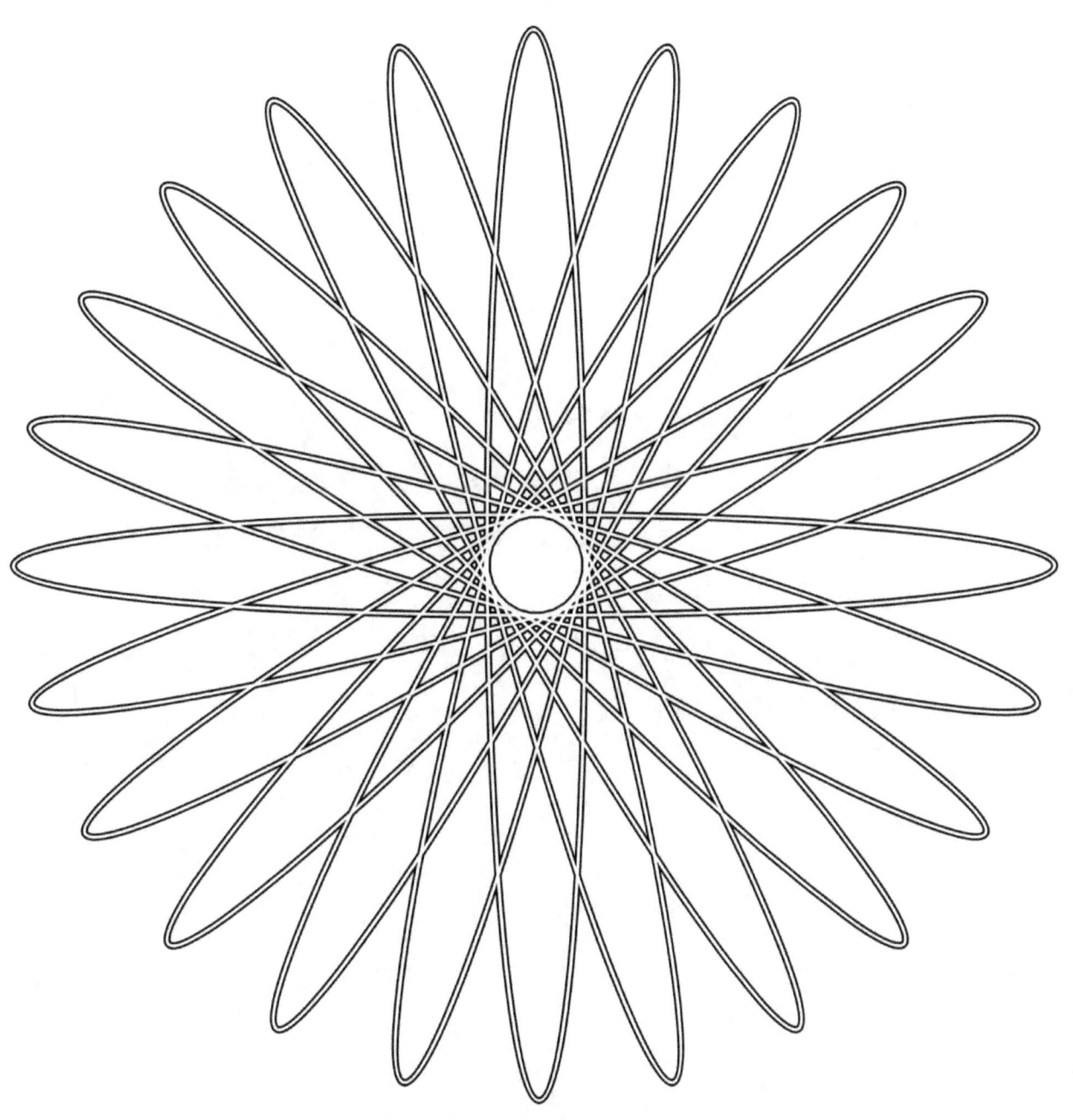

If you end up with a boring, miserable life because you listened to your mom, your dad, your teacher, your priest, or some guy on television telling you how to do your shit, then you deserve it.

Frank Zappa

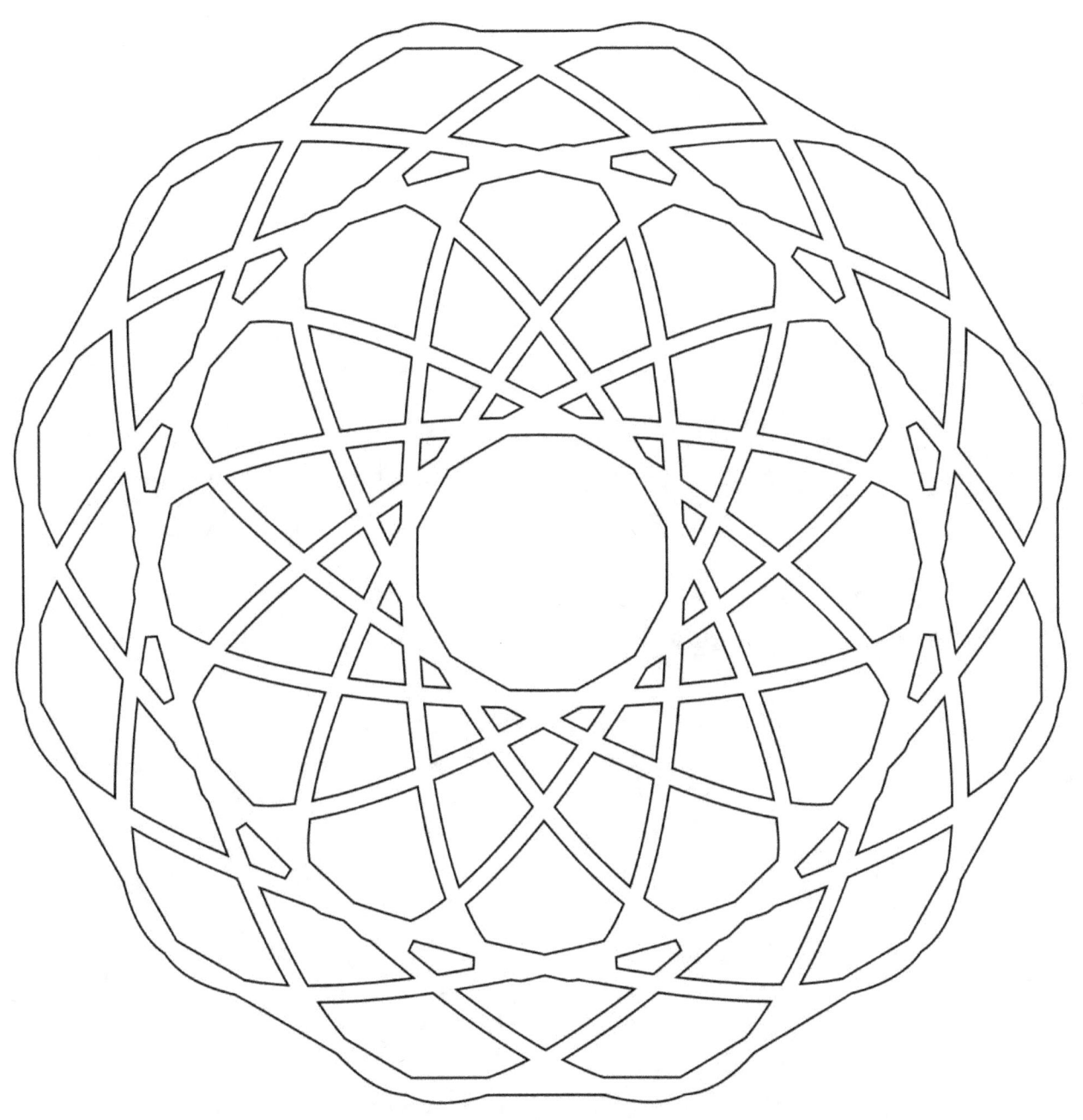

If you don't design your own life plan, chances are you'll fall into someone else's plan.
And guess what they have planned for you? Not much.

Unknown

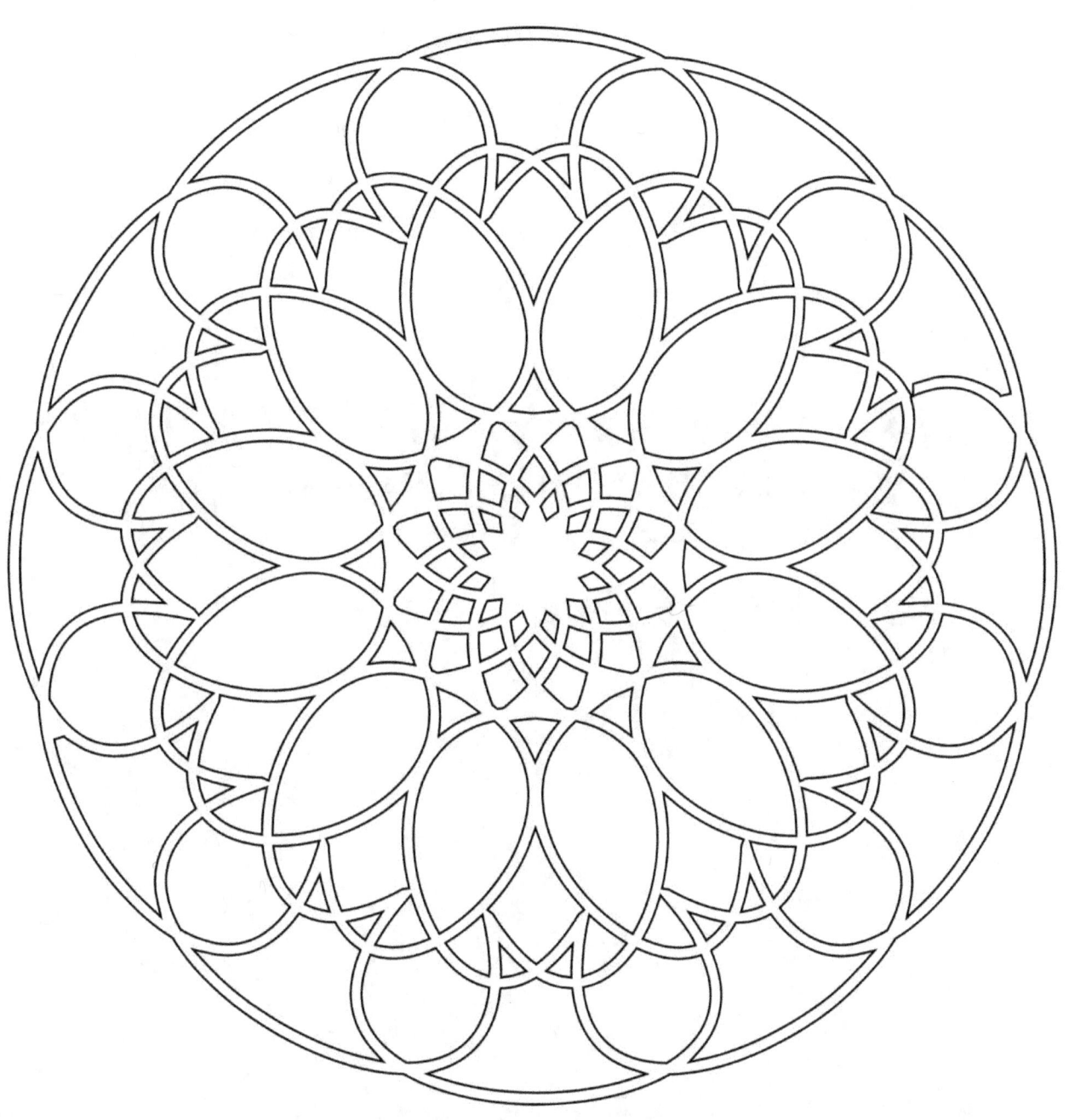

I have a simple philosophy: Fill what's empty. Empty what's full. Scratch where it itches.

Alice Roosevelt Longworth

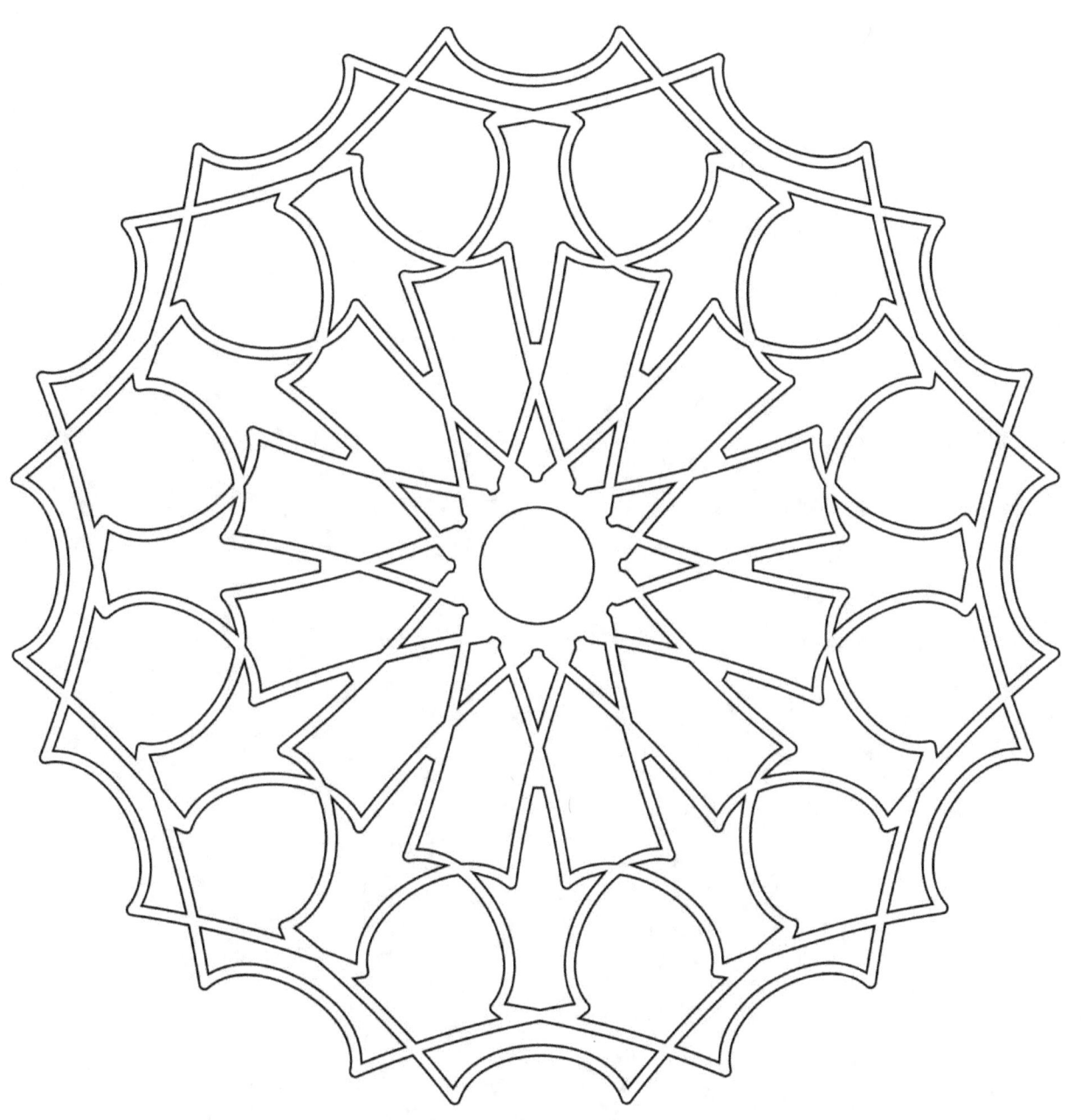

Life is a shipwreck but we must not forget to sing in the lifeboats.

Voltaire

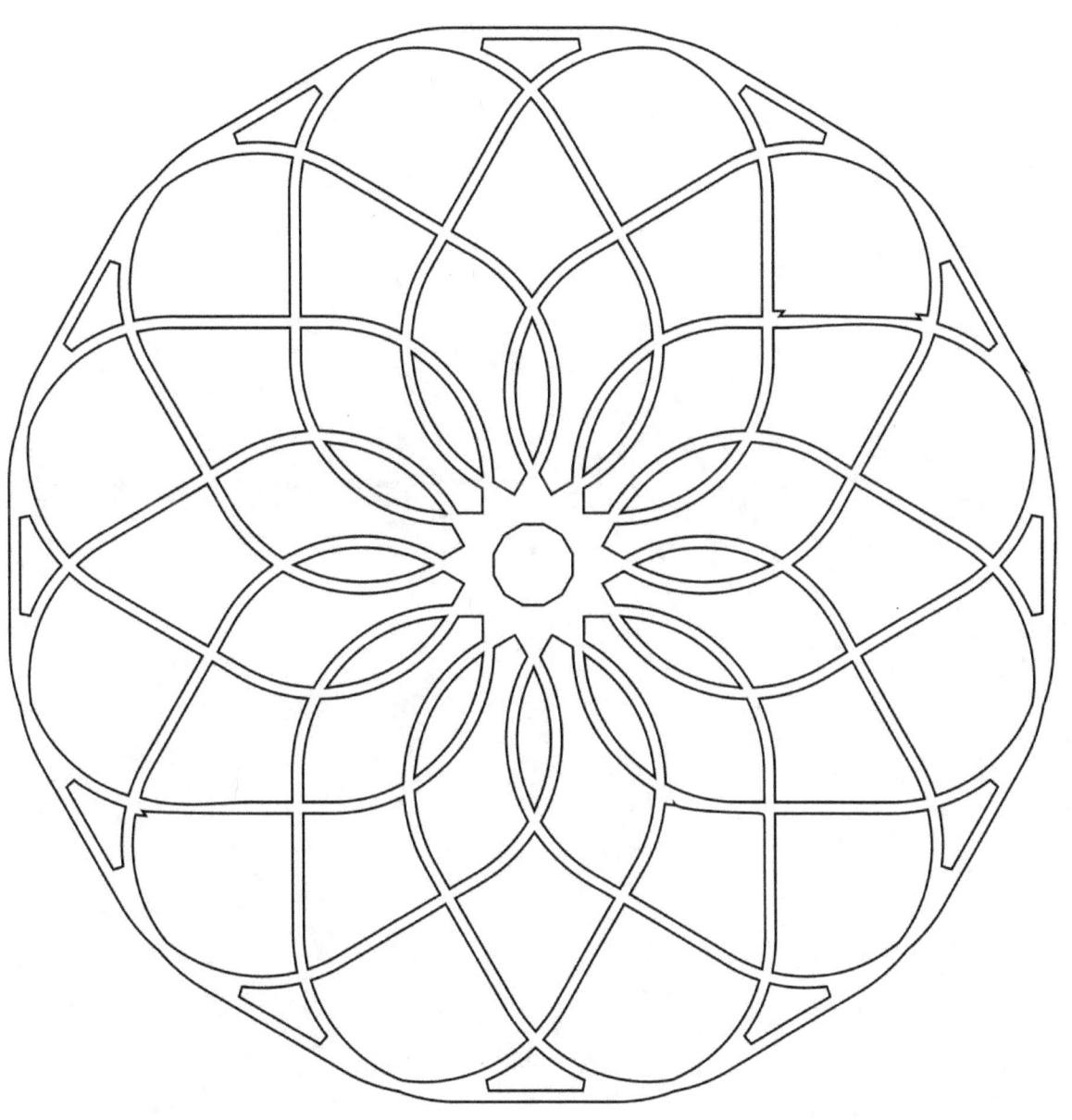

I didn't fail the test. I just found 100 ways to do it wrong.

Benjamin Franklin

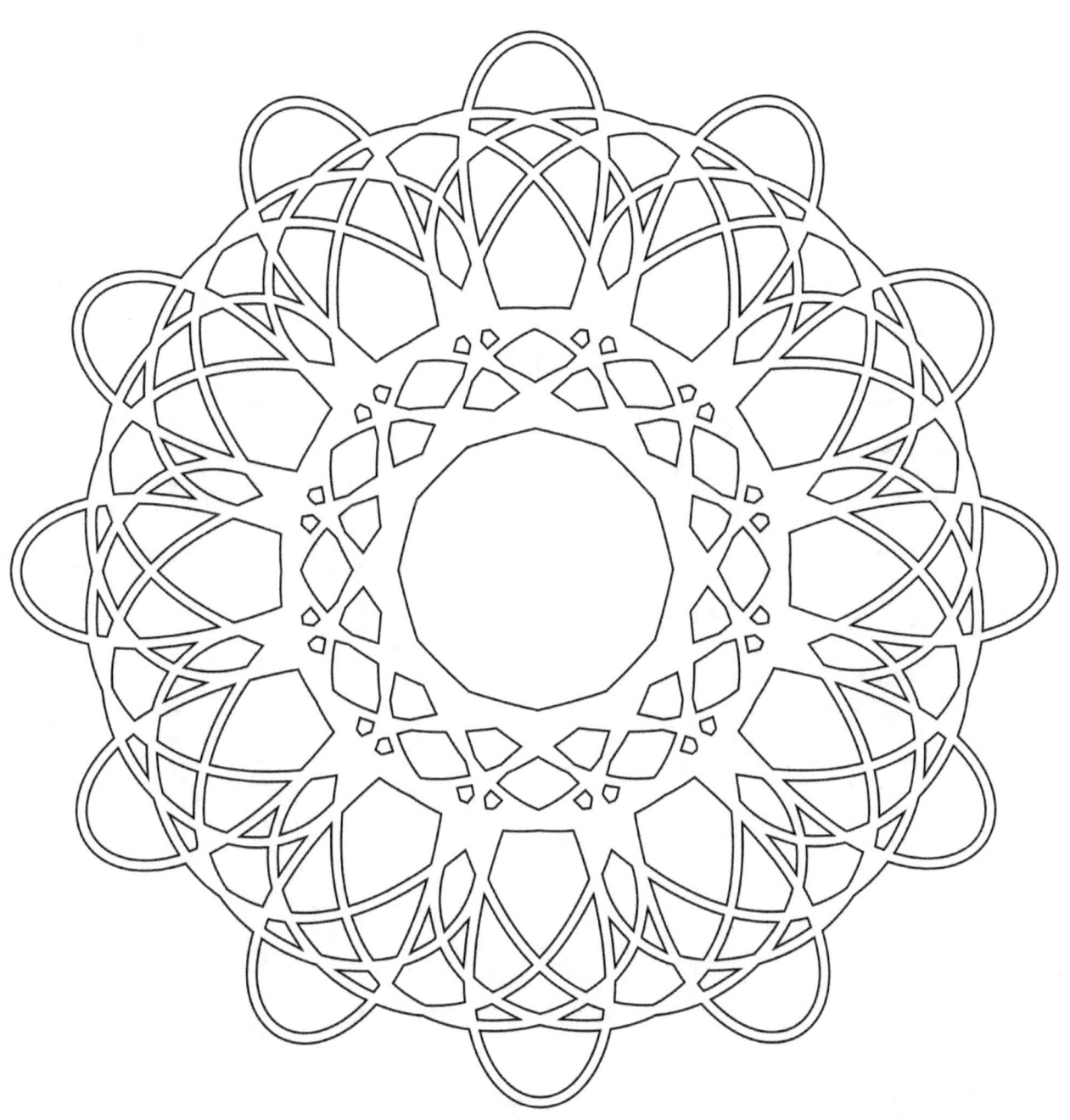

**Consider the postage stamp:
its usefulness consists in the ability
to stick to one thing 'til it gets there.**
Josh Billings

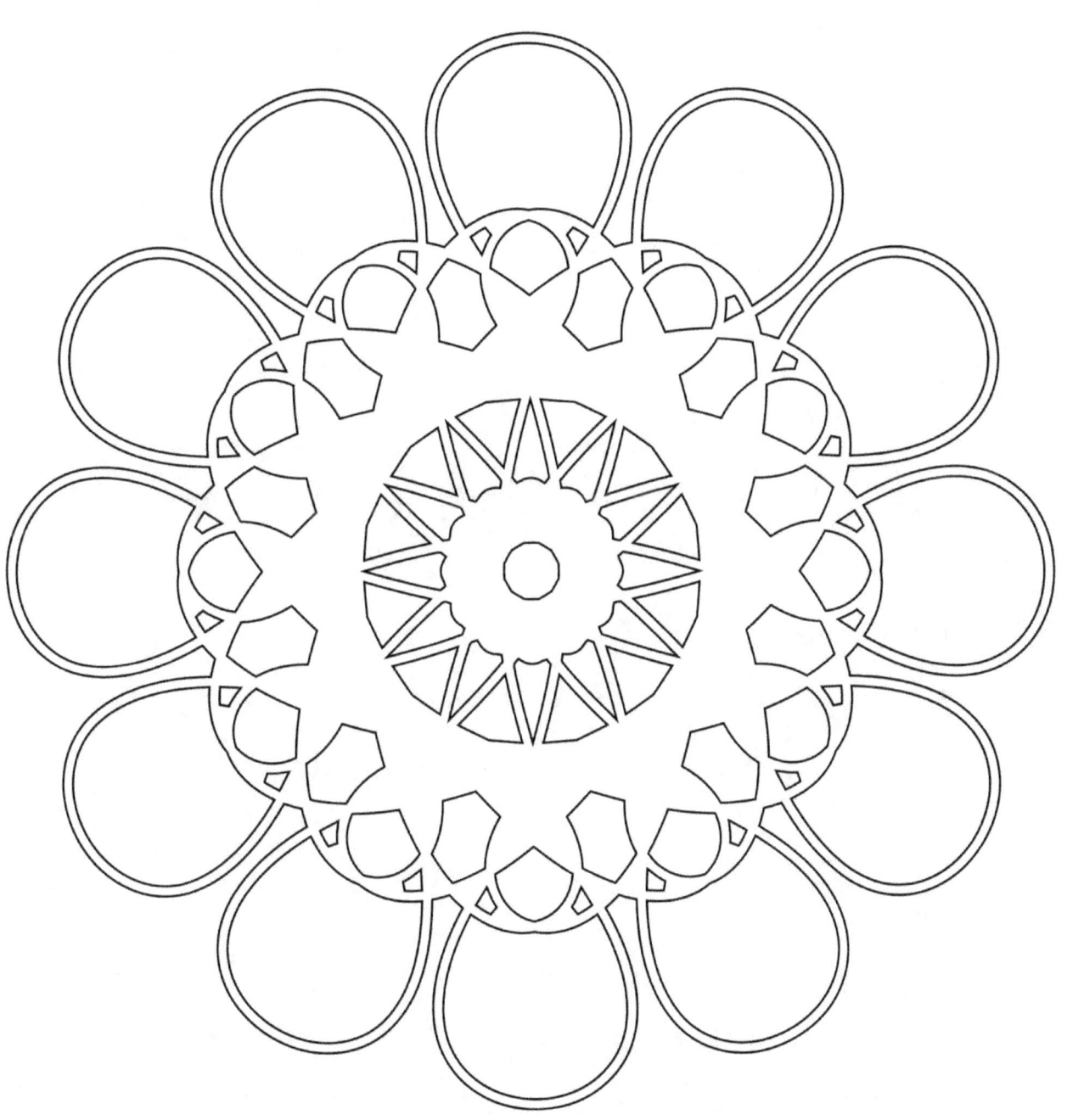

When life gives you lemons, squirt someone in the eye.

Cathy Guisewite

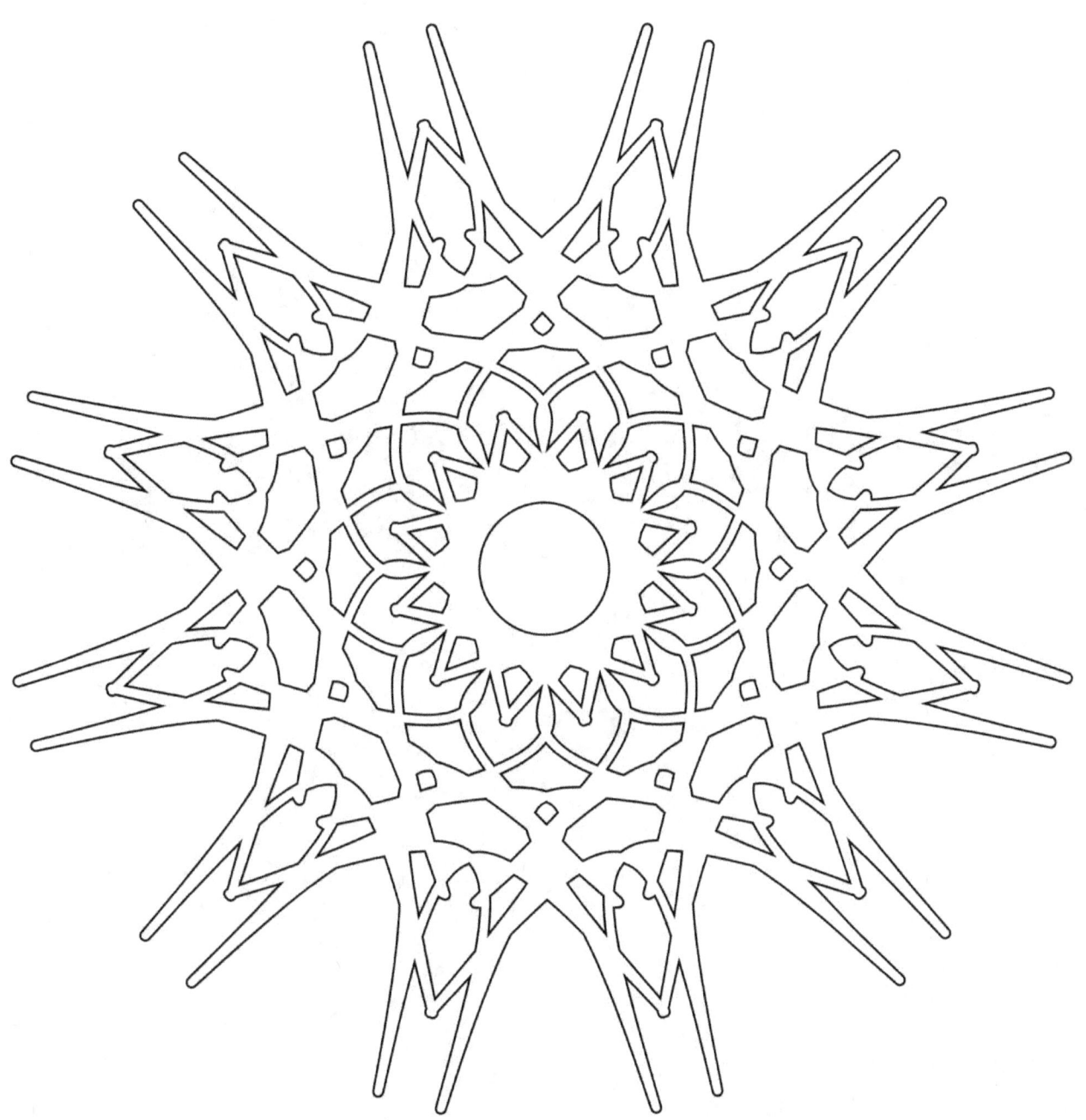

Good things come to those who wait... greater things come to those who get off their ass and do anything to make it happen.

Unknown

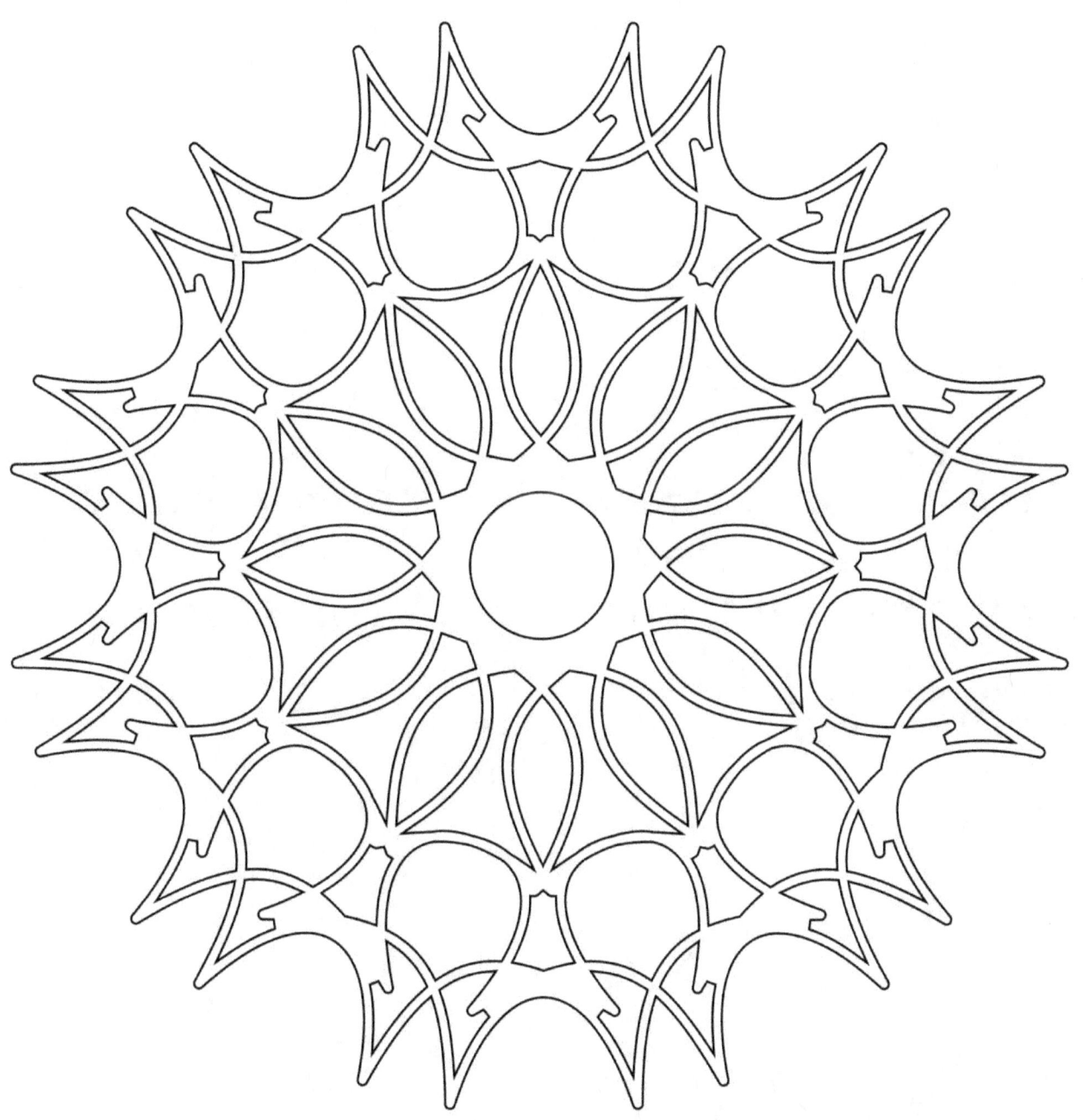

**Don't worry about the world coming to an end today.
It's already tomorrow in Australia.**

Charles Schulz

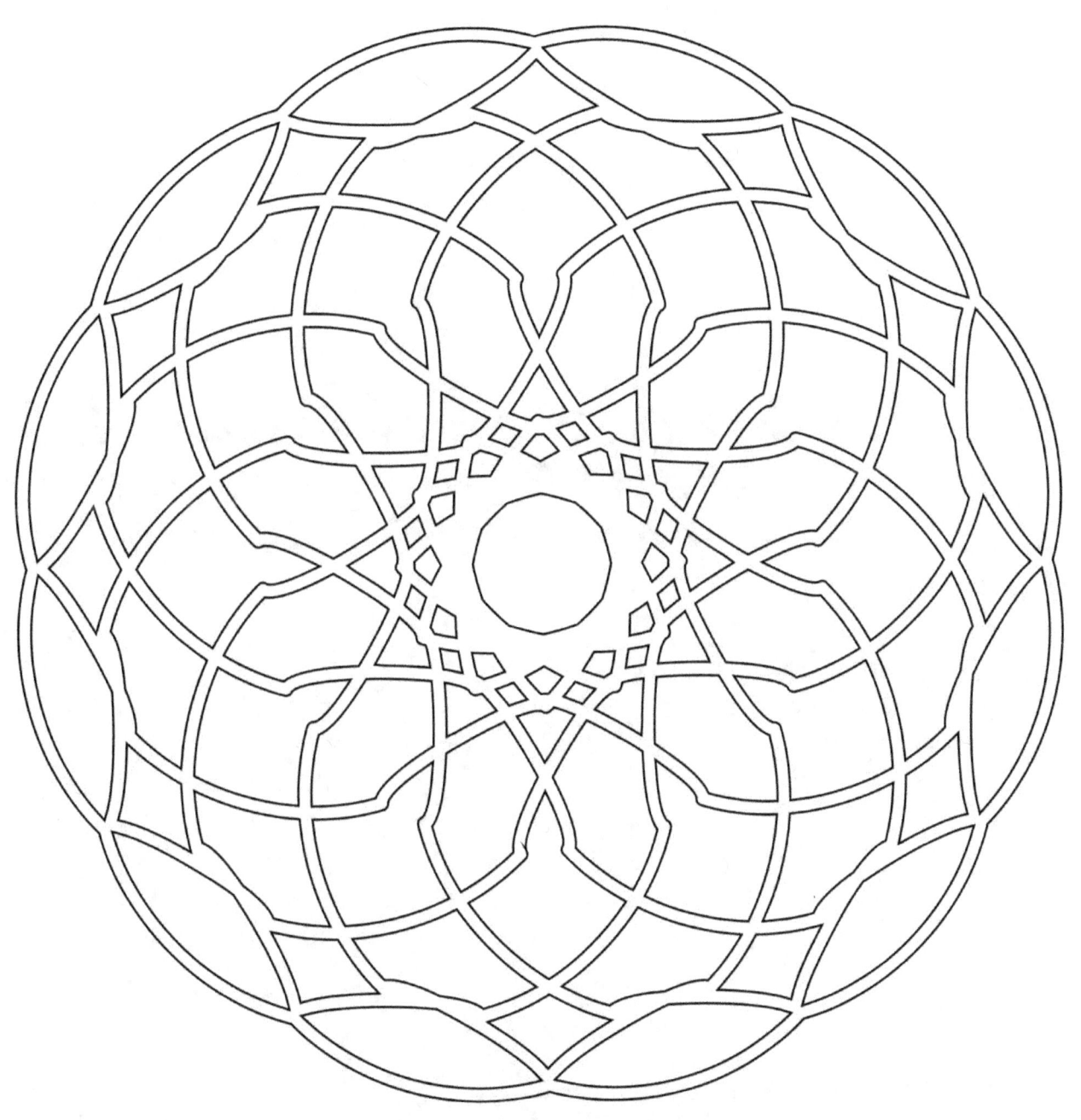

Edison failed 10, 000 times before he made the electric light.
Do not be discouraged if you fail a few times.

Napoleon Hill

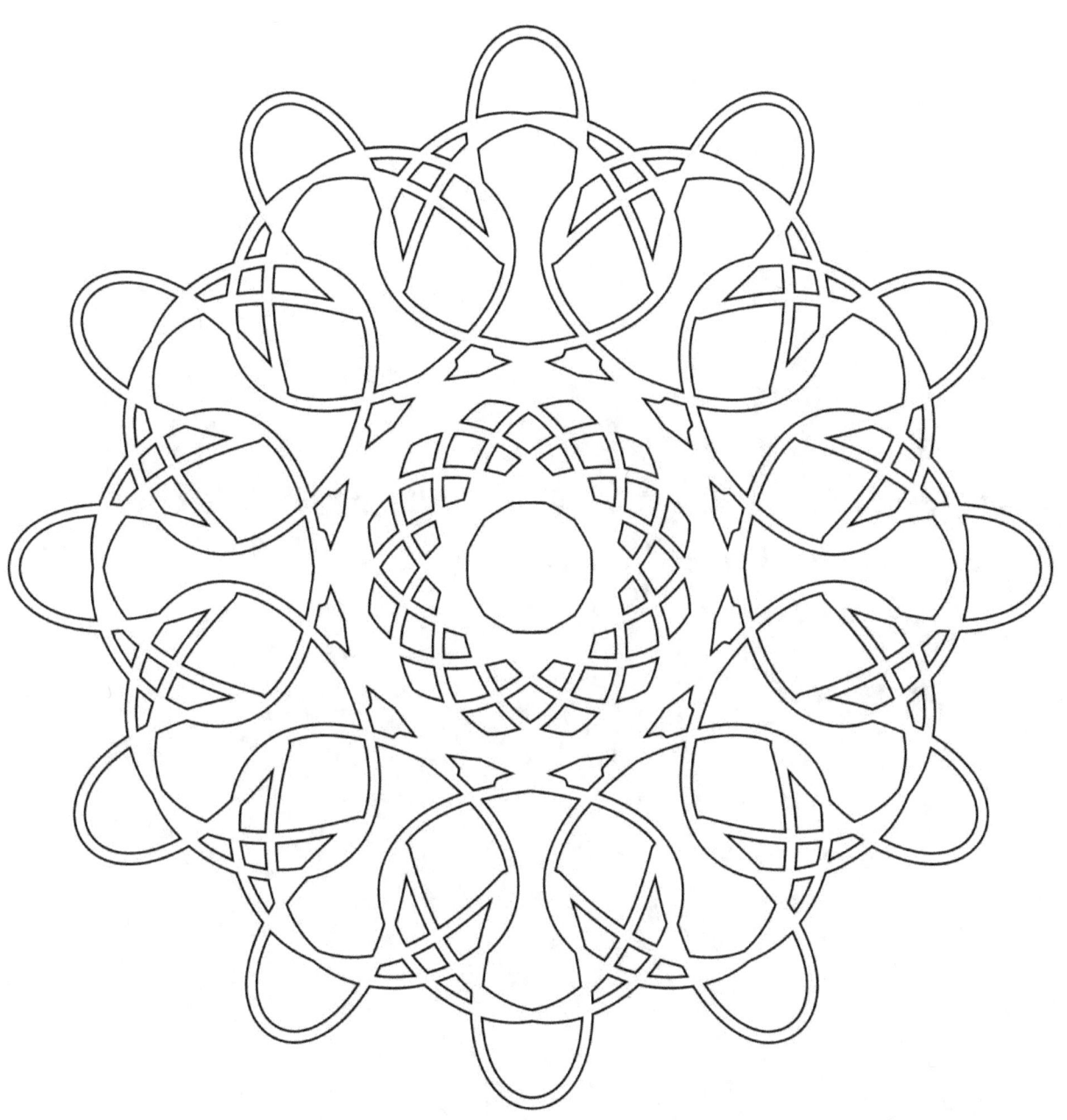

Here is a test to find whether your mission on earth is finished: If you're alive it isn't.

Richard Bach

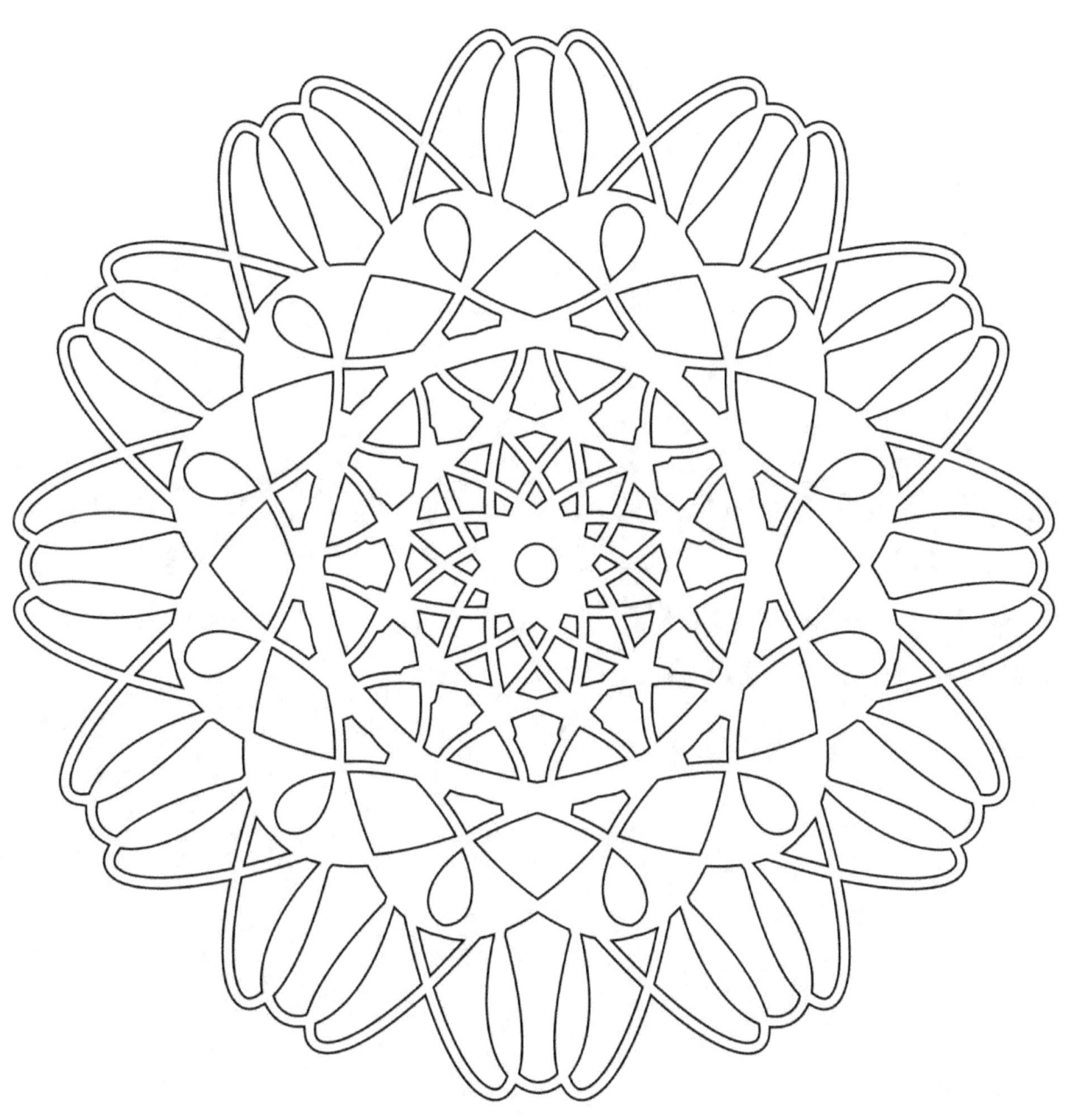

I'll probably never fully become what I wanted to be when I grew up, but that's probably because I wanted to be a ninja princess.

Cassandra Duffy

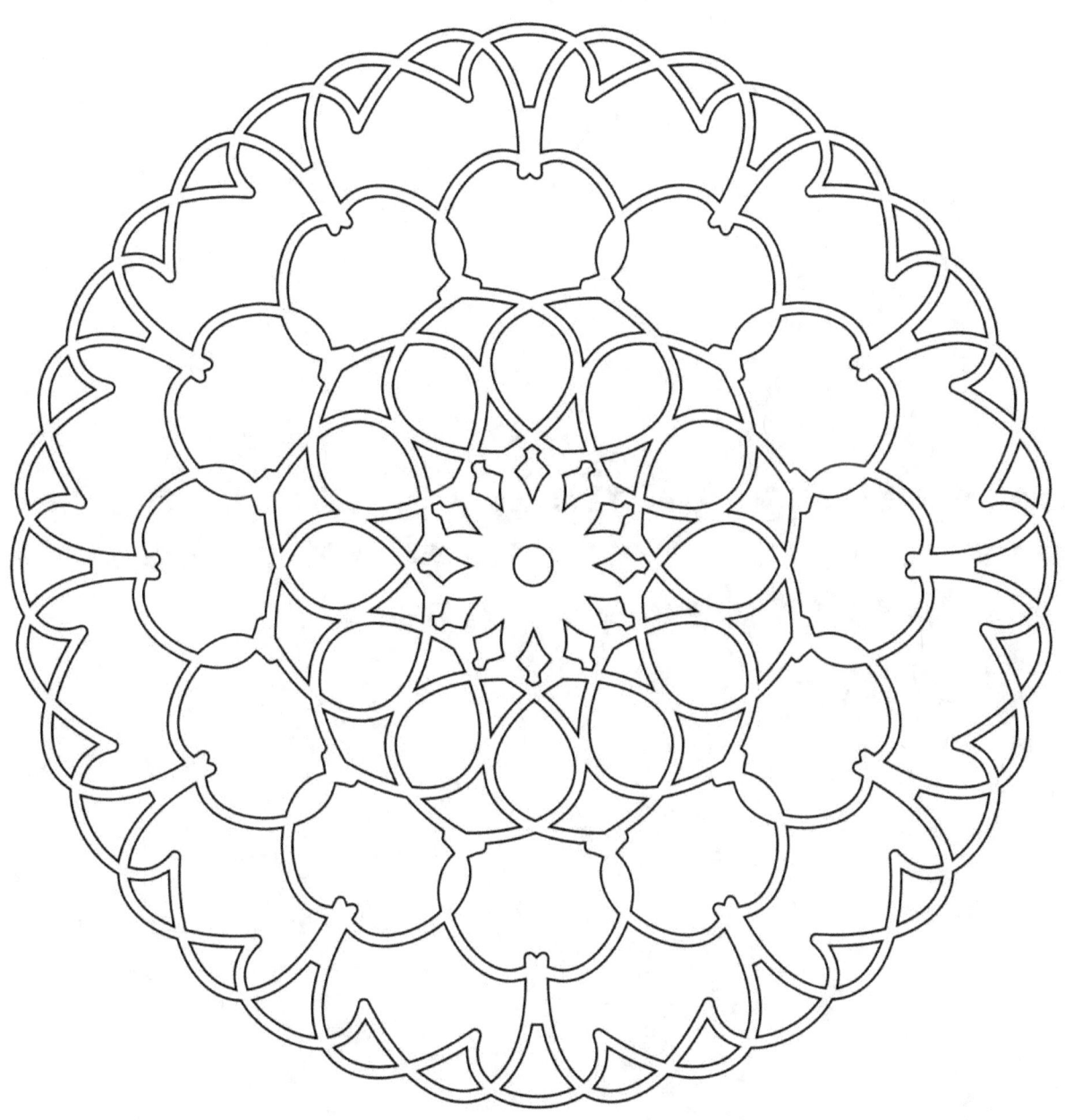

By working faithfully eight hours a day you may eventually get to be boss and work twelve hours a day.

Robert Frost

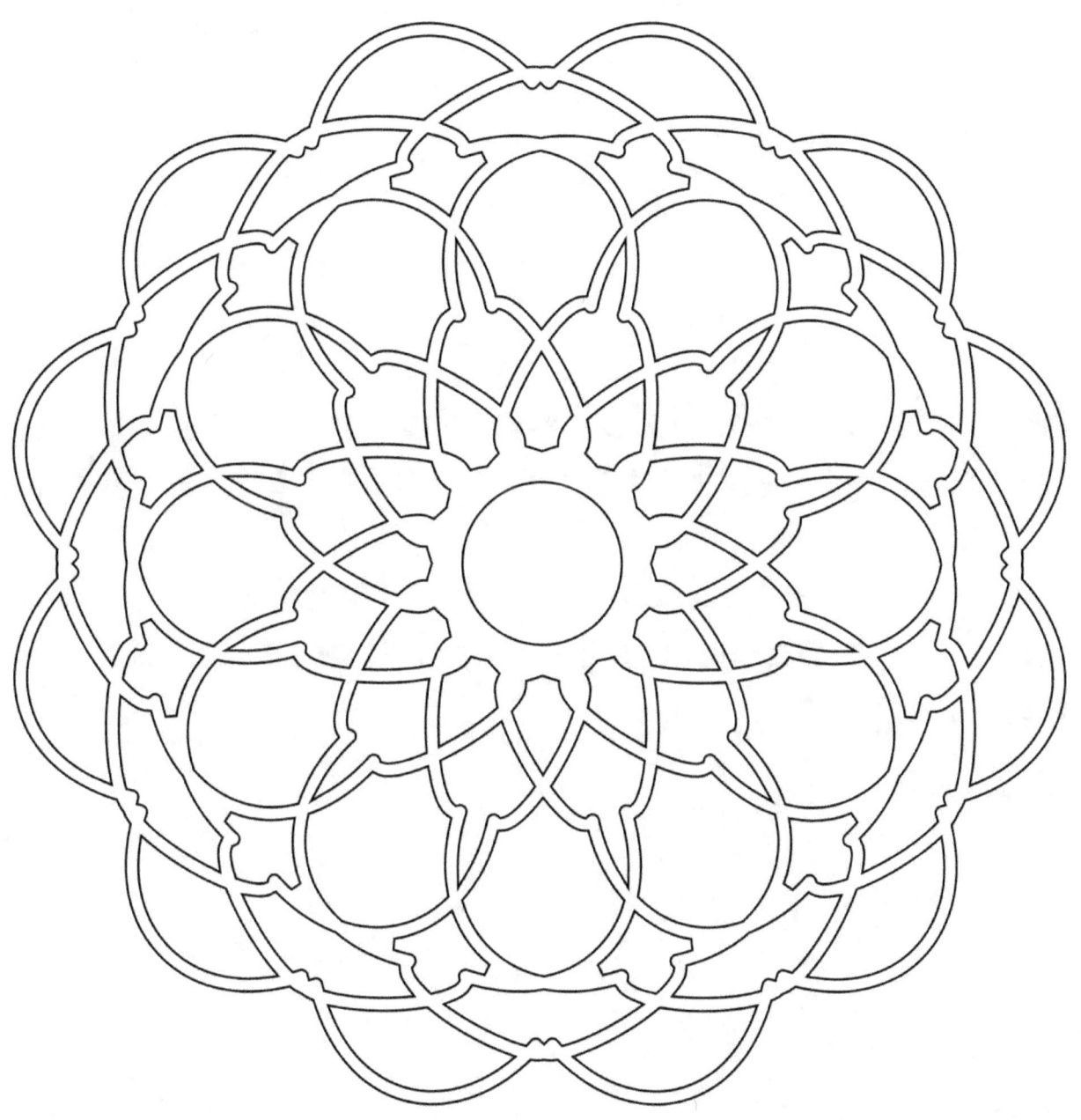

My therapist told me the way to achieve true inner peace is to finish what I start.
So far I've finished two bags of M&Ms and a chocolate cake. I feel better already.

Dave Barry

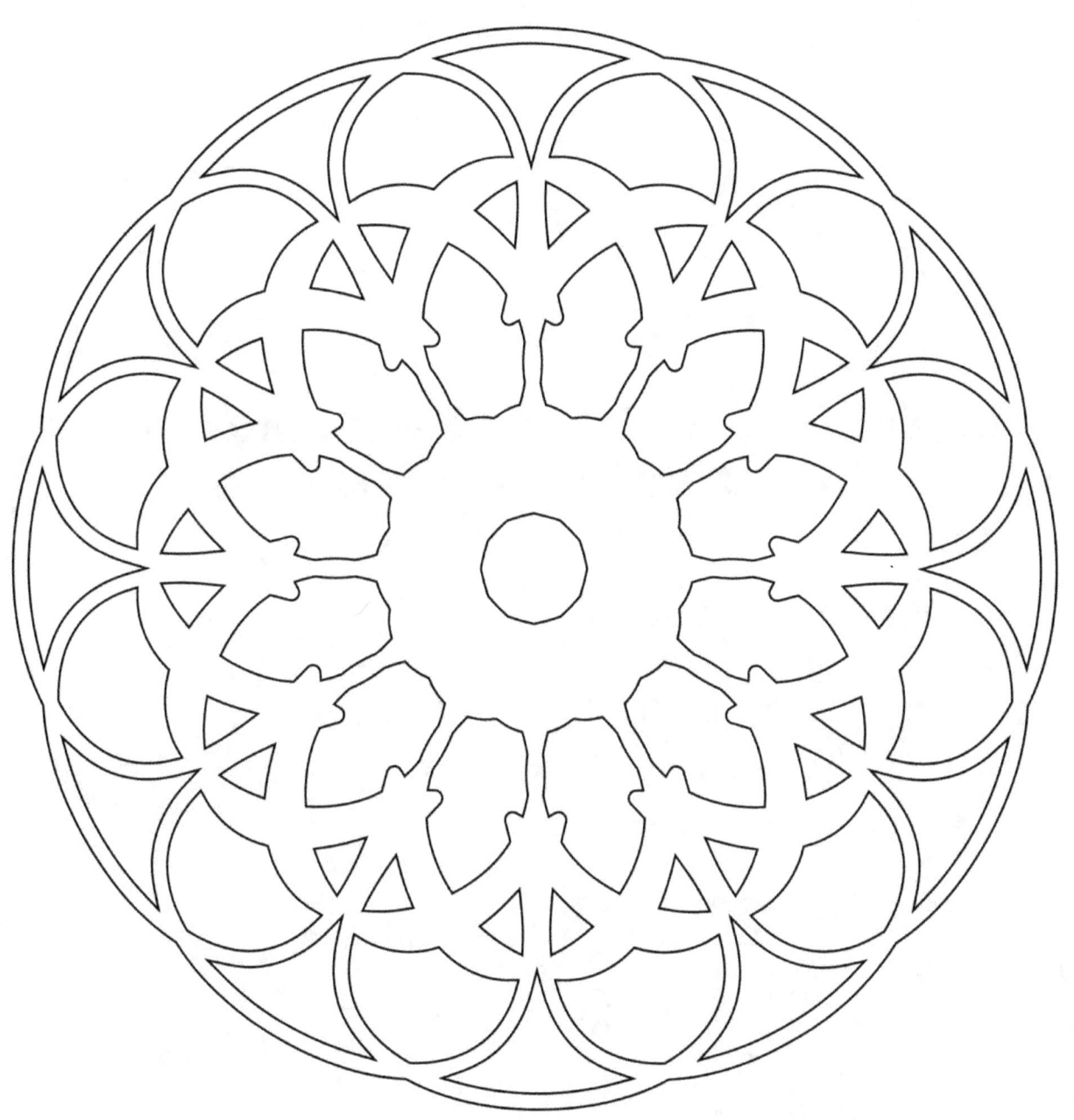

Whoever said, 'It's not whether you win or lose that counts,' probably lost.

Martina Navratilova

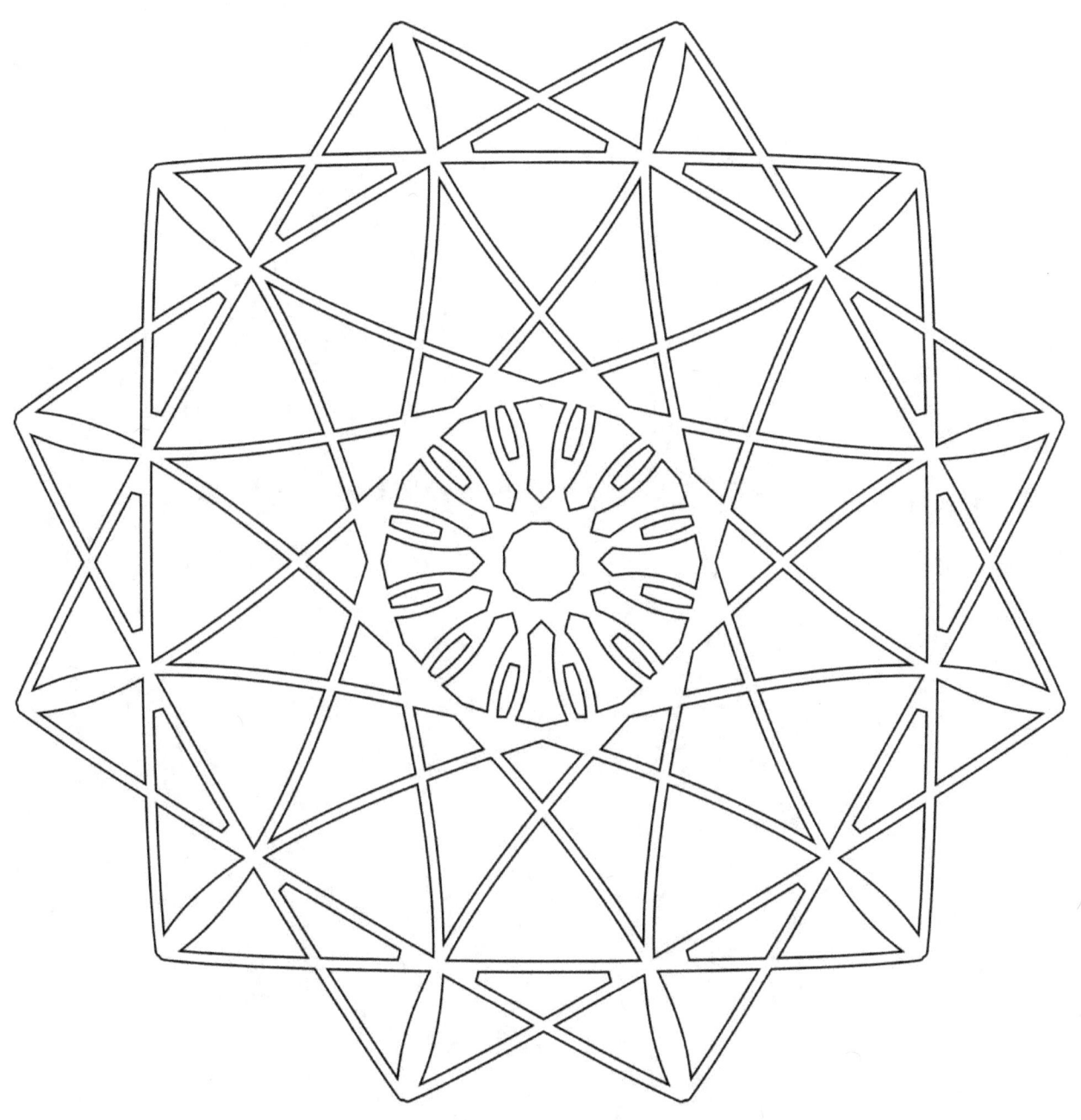

If you fall, I'll always be there.

The Floor

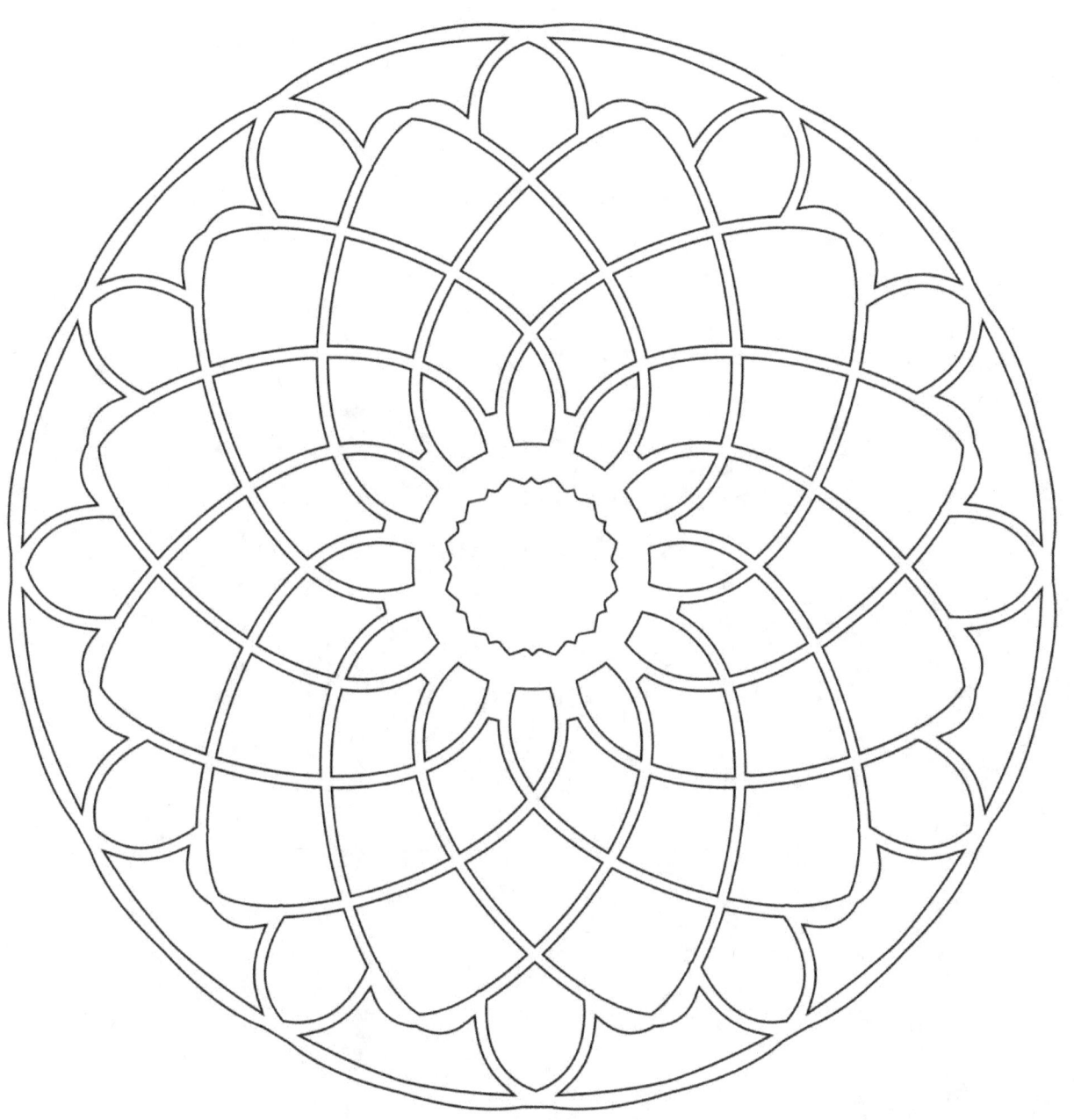

**Focus, focus, focus!
What am I, a telescope?!**

Naruto Uzumaki

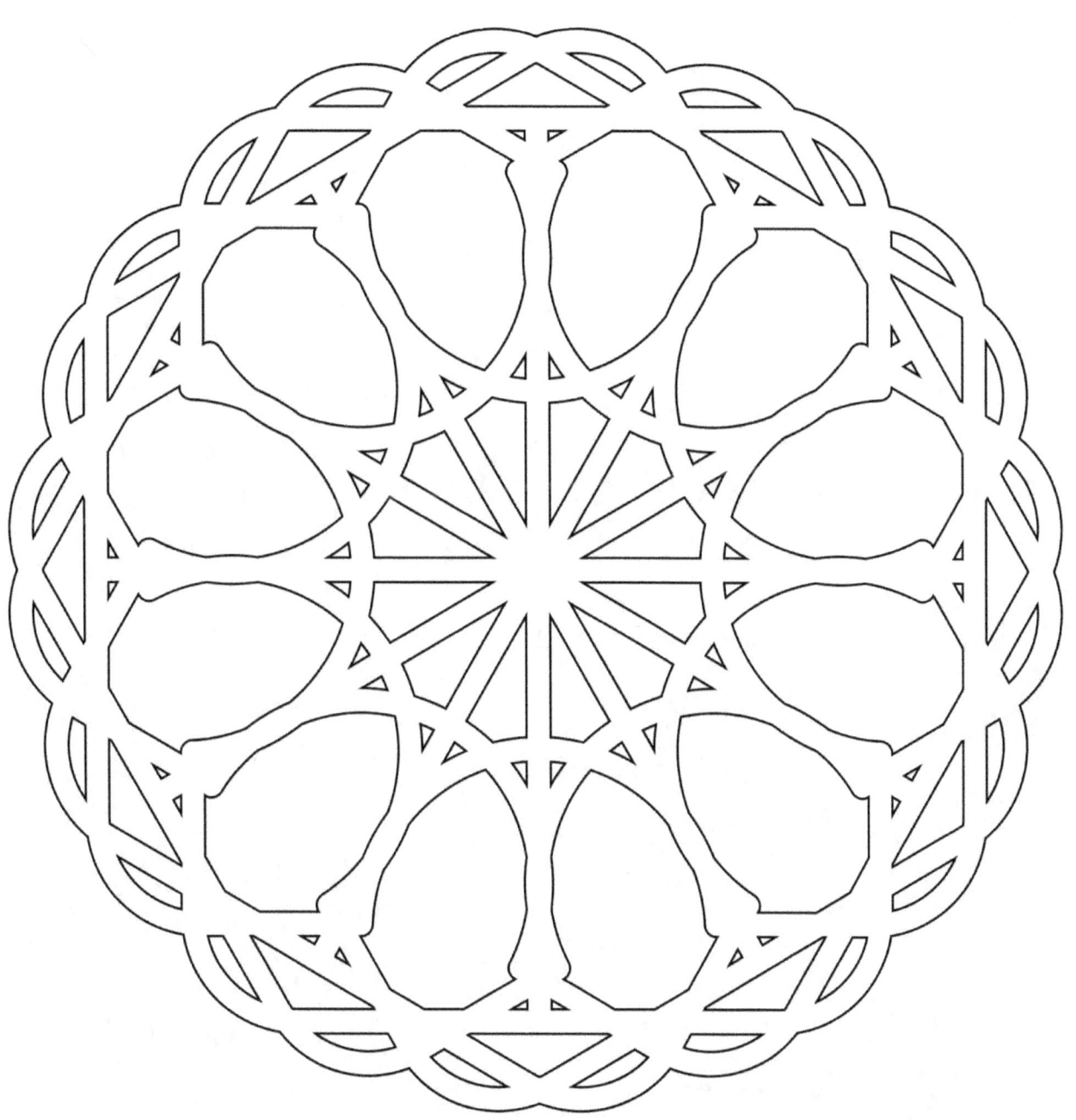

**I intend to live forever.
So far, so good.**

Steven Wright

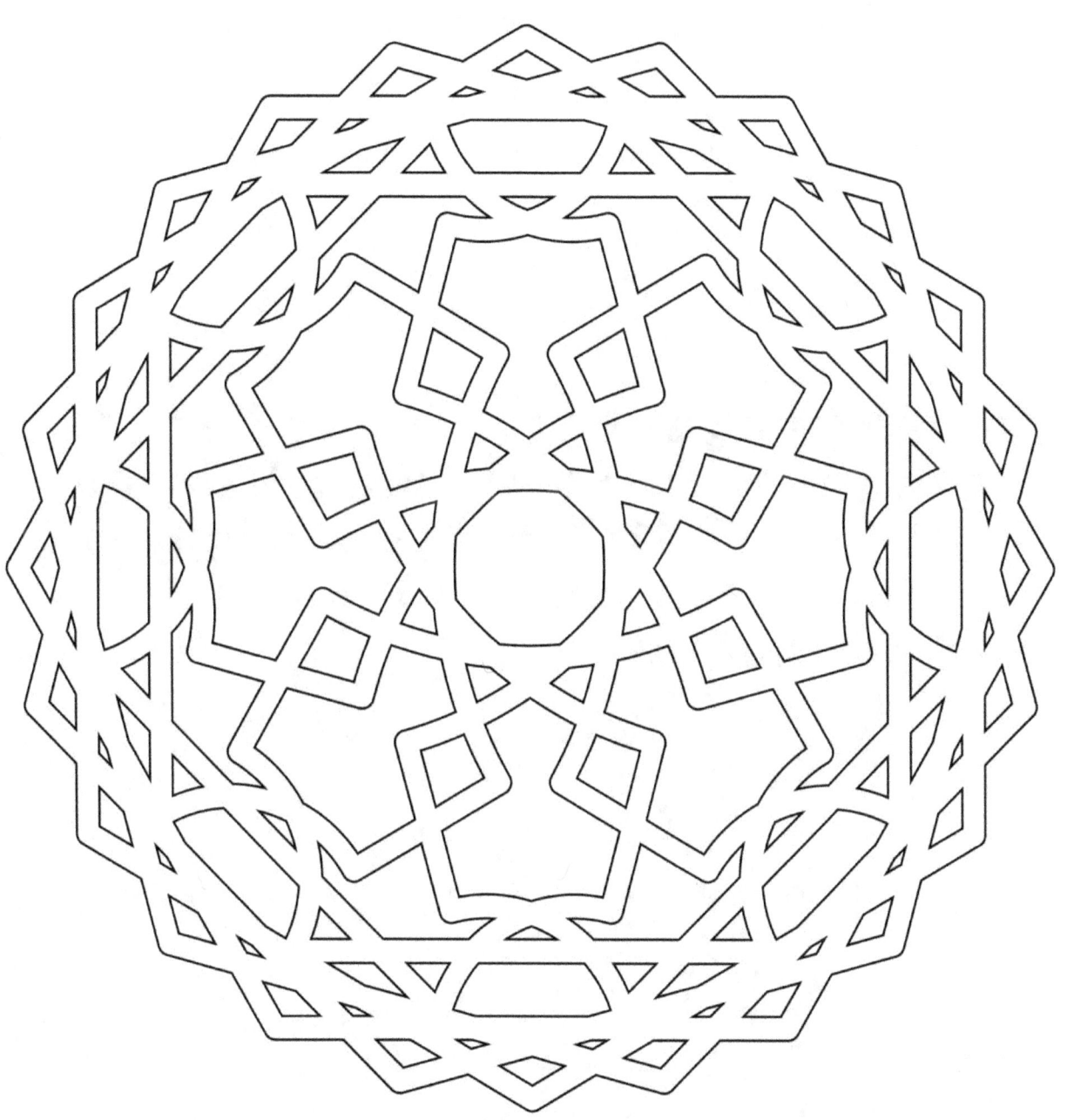

Sometimes you climb out of bed in the morning and you think, "I'm not going to make it." But you laugh inside – remembering all the times you felt that way.

Charles Bukowski

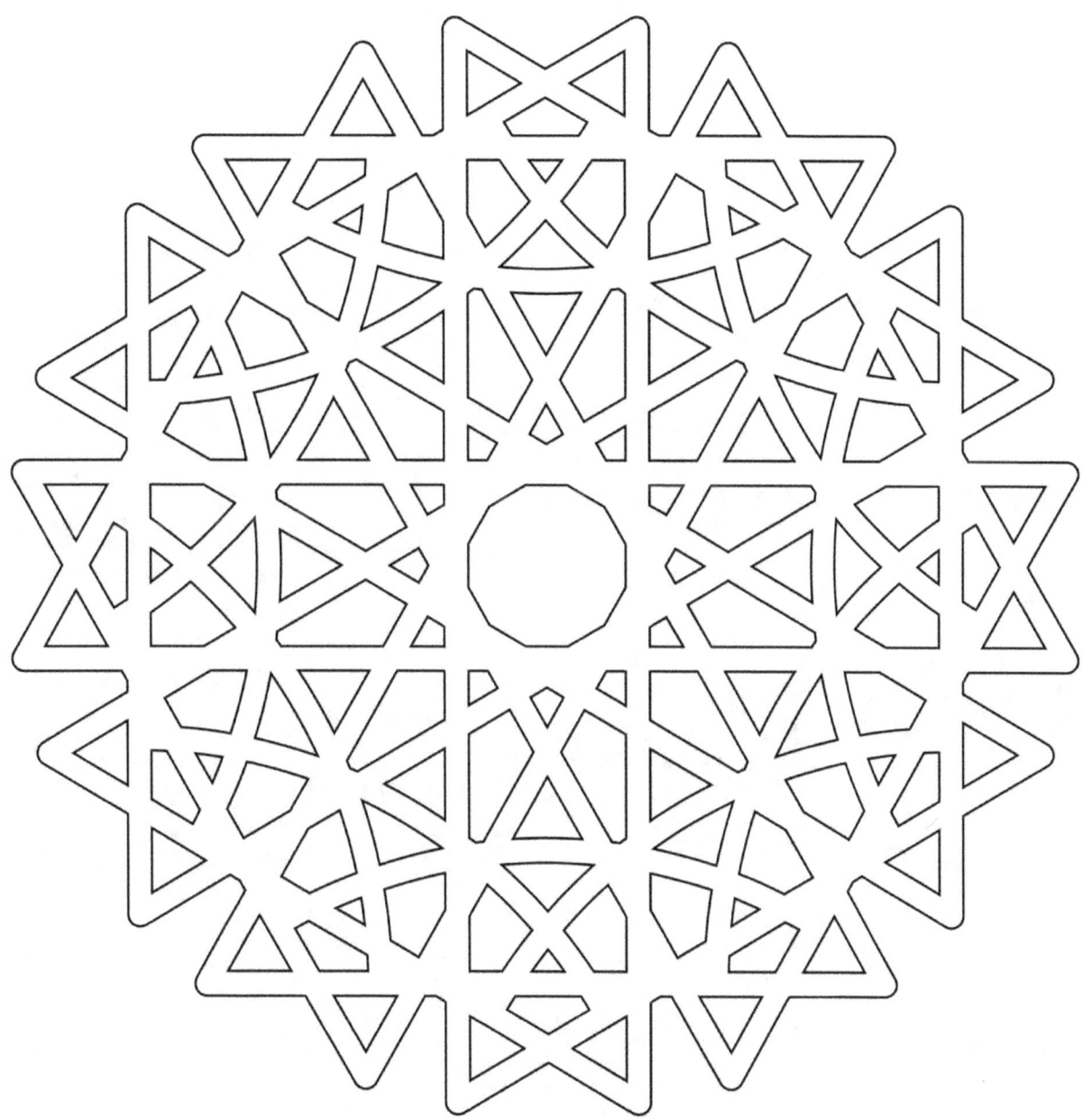

**Accept who you are.
Unless you are a serial killer, that is.**

Ellen Dejeneres

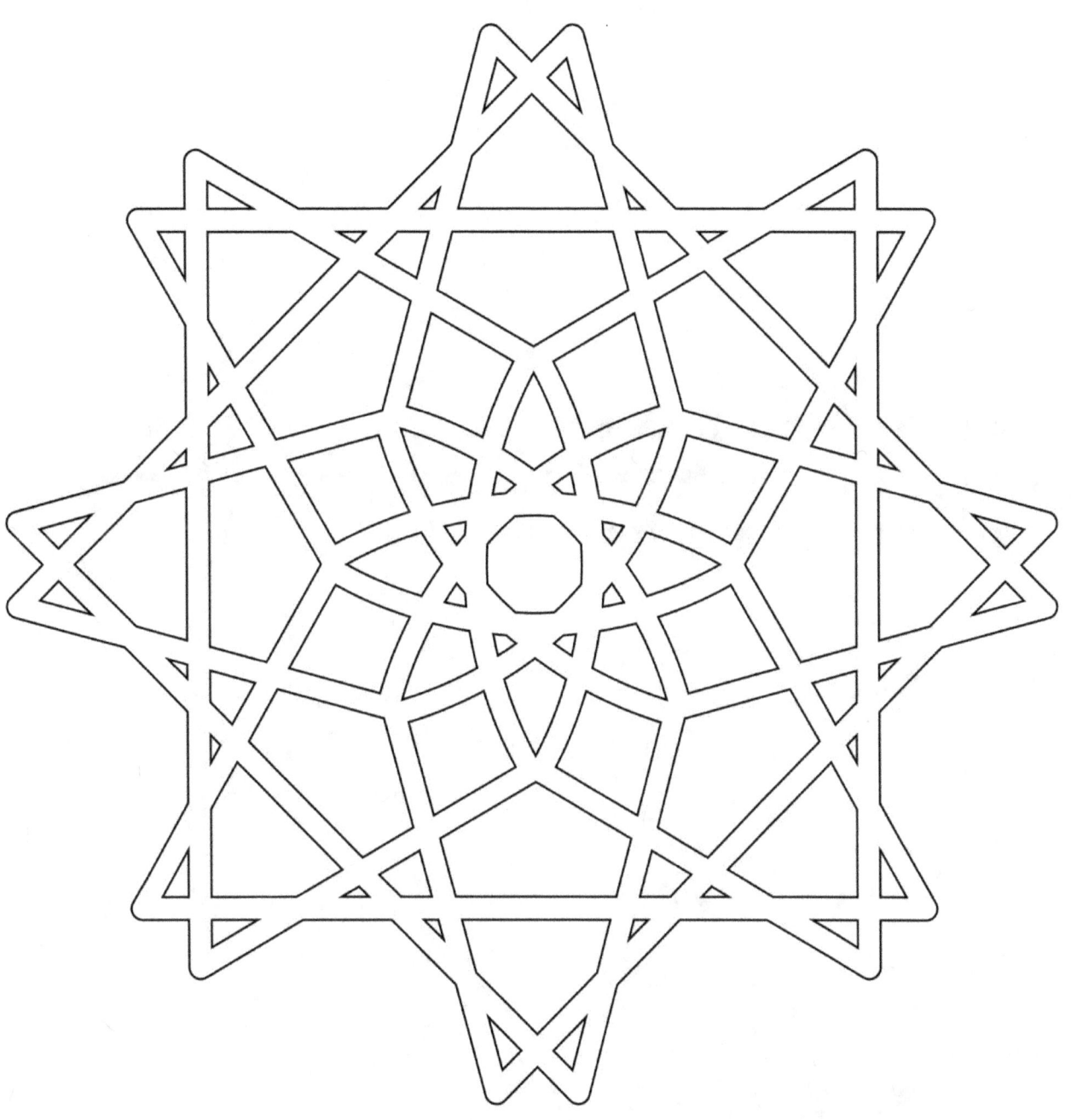

The elevator to success is out of order- you'll have to take the stairs... One step at a time.

Joe Girard

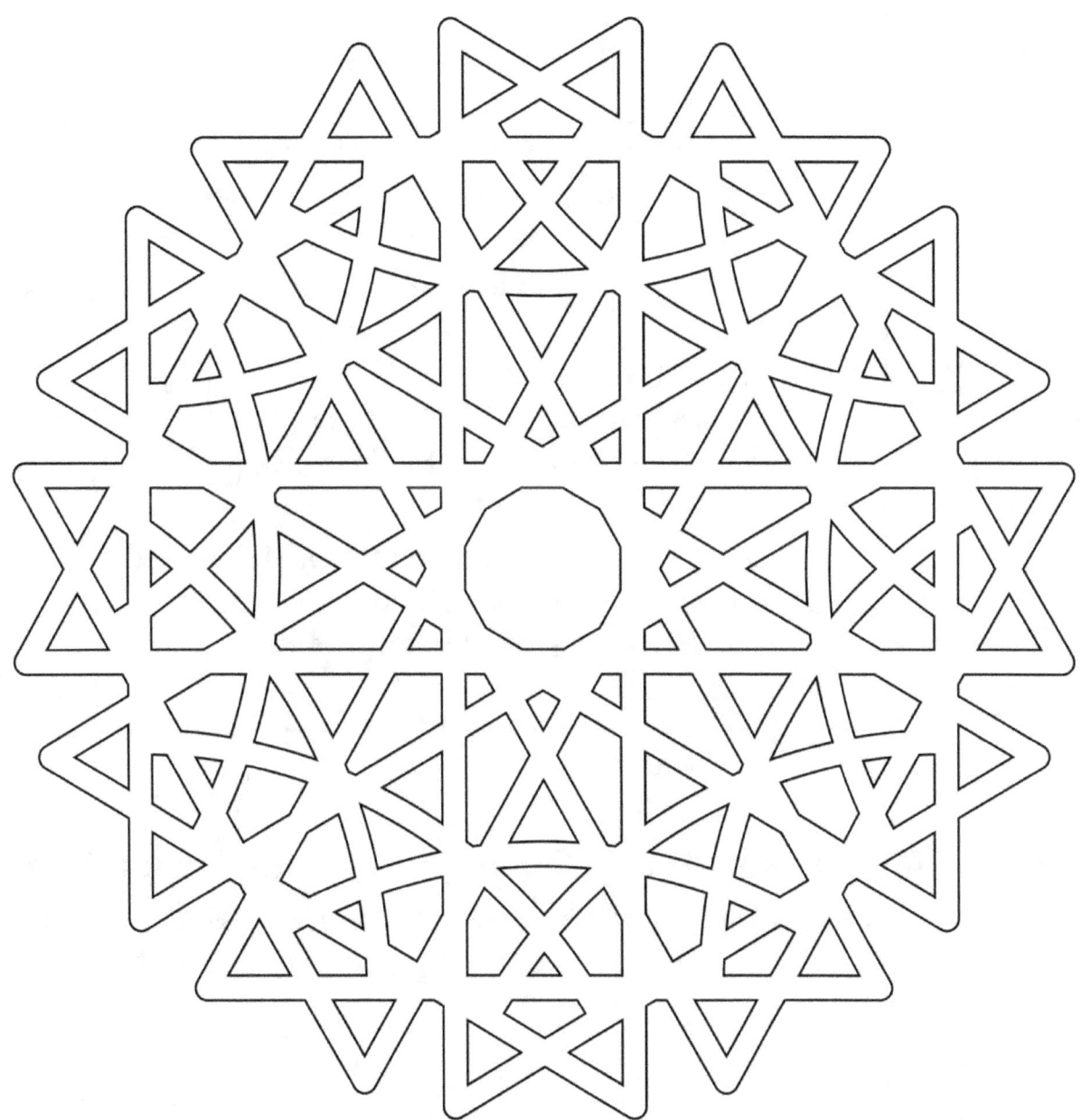

DON'T FORGET

Register and get your **FREE**
pdf of **Coloring Pages**
At: www.DancingWithYourLife.com
And check out the full range of
our books and products while you're there.

ALSO

Email us a photo of your proudest colored page
from one of our coloring books to:
support@DancingWithYourLife.com

The best ones selected each month will be posted
on our web site and these **winners will get their
choice of a free coloring book**

And to help others who may be considering this book,
please share your experience with a brief review at:
www.amazon.com/gp/product/994423047